HEALTHCARE CAREER GUIDE

companion book with HEALTHCARE CAREER GUIDE

Susan Odegaard Turner, RN PhD

JULY 2013

TABLE OF CONTENTS

HEALTHCARE CAREER GUIDE

Instructor Guide Chapter 1

SUGGESTED TEACHING
TECHNIQUES:

1. Small group discussions
2. Classroom discussion questions
3. Individual completion of
   Self-assessment tools
4. Resources List

EACH CHAPTER INCLUDES:

- Learning objectives
- Chapter key concepts
- Discussion questions:
- Case studies

CHAPTER 1. HEALTHCARE AS A CAREER

Chapter Objectives:

1. Discuss and identify components of the healthcare delivery system.

2. Discuss economic impact of healthcare jobs.

3. List 5 occupations within healthcare.

4. List two occupations that require an advanced degree.

5. List two jobs that do not require a college degree.

6. Identify 63 trends in healthcare industry within the next ten-twenty years.

7. Identify 5 qualities healthcare workers should possess

Overview of Healthcare Industry

- Healthcare provided 14.3 million jobs for wage and salary workers, according to the Bureau of Labor Statistics (bls.gov).

- Currently, even in a tepid economy, ten of the 20 fastest growing occupations are healthcare related (bls.gov).

- Healthcare will generate 3.2 million new wage and salary jobs between 2008 and 2018, more than any other industry, largely in response to rapid growth in the elderly population.

- Healthcare jobs can be found throughout the country, but they are concentrated in metropolitan areas.

- Employment in the healthcare industry is projected to increase 22 percent through 2018, compared with 11 percent for all industries combined (bls.gov) (table 3).

- Healthcare firms employ large numbers of workers in professional and service occupations. Together, these two occupational groups account for 76 percent of jobs in the industry (table 2).

- Healthcare combines medical technology and human interaction to diagnose, treat, and provide care around the clock, responding to the needs of millions of people

- A wide variety of people with various educational backgrounds are necessary for the healthcare industry to function.

- Professional occupations, such as physicians and surgeons, dentists, registered nurses, social workers, and physical therapists, usually require at least a bachelor's degree in a specialized field or higher education in a specific health field, although registered nurses also may enter through associate degree programs.

- Health technologists and technicians can operate medical equipment and assist a variety of practitioners with diagnosis and/or treatment. These healthcare workers typically attend 1-year or 2-year postsecondary (after high school) training programs. (bls.gov)

- Healthcare service occupations can also attract many workers with minimal or no specialized education or training. Some of these workers are nursing aides, home health aides, building maintenance and cleaning workers, dental assistants, medical assistants, and personal and home care aides.

Education and Training

- A variety of postsecondary programs provide specialized training for jobs in the healthcare industry. People interested in a career as a diagnosing and treating practitioner—such as physicians and surgeons, optometrists, physical therapists, advanced practice nurses or audiologists—should be prepared to complete graduate school coupled with years of education beyond college.

- A few healthcare workers need bachelor's degrees like social workers, health service managers, and some registered nurses. A majority of the technologist and technician occupations require a certificate or an associate degree; these programs usually have both classroom and clinical instruction and last about 2 years. Many can be obtained at local community colleges or vocational/technical schools.

- Many hospitals provide training, tuition assistance, or advancement in return for a promise to work at their facility in that role for a particular length of time after graduation.

- Healthcare workers at all levels of education and training will continue to be in demand.

- Average earnings of nonsupervisory workers in most healthcare segments are higher than the average for all private industry, with hospital workers earning considerably more than the average and those employed in nursing and residential care facilities and home healthcare services earning less .

- Healthcare is an excellent second career option

Should you consider a Healthcare career?

Persons considering careers in healthcare should have:

- A strong desire to help others, genuine concern for the welfare of patients.

- An ability to deal with people of diverse backgrounds in stressful situations.

- A love for Science

- Commitment to Life Long Learning

- Comfort in a Health Care Setting

- Ability to deal with a wide variety of people

- Ability to work collaboratively as a Team Player

- There are numerous other health-related work settings that do not require direct patient contact.

Discussion Questions:

1. Discuss pros and cons of direct patient care jobs.

2. Identify healthcare trends over ten to twenty years.

3. Identify components of healthcare system.

4. Compare and contrast professional healthcare roles, education and expectations.

5. Compare and contrast professional healthcare roles, education and expectations.

Case Studies:

1. Eleanor is a single mother of three small children. She has worked in retail sales until her recent layoff. She is 33 years old. What healthcare careers might she consider? How can she finance any needed education?

2. Fred is a computer programmer who has lost his job twice in 3 years. He knows there has been recent legislation about electronic medical records. He asks your opinion on a healthcare career in this area of specialty. What do you tell him and why?

LIFE AS A NEW HEALTHCARE GRADUATE

Instructor Guide
Chapter 2

CHAPTER 2. LIFE AS A NEW HEALTHCARE WORKER

Chapter Objectives:

1. Identify the process for certification or licensure in your new role.

2. Explain the concept of a novice in healthcare.

3. List 5 things to consider when making your first job selection.

4. Explain the concept of life/work balance, and its importance.

Key terms

Licensure	Preceptor
Certification	New graduate program
Interim permit	Life balance
Job offer	Courtesy
Interview	
Orientation	

Key concepts: Your License

- Most professional healthcare roles require either certification or licensure.

- The process for each healthcare specialty varies by state and healthcare specialty.

- Interim permits allow nursing school graduates to work as IPs while waiting to take their nursing exams and waiting for their license.

- When you obtain your license or certificate, you are a graduate healthcare worker in your specialty.

- You are entering the healthcare profession as a novice, or someone who has education, but little or no experience.

Your First Healthcare Job after Graduation

- Many new grads in healthcare professions know before they take their state licensing exams or certification tests where they will be working once they finish school.

- Most hospitals offer new graduates jobs as soon as students have finished school.

- You must marketing yourself as a new grad/new worker

- Don't make a quick decision and accept a position after a first interview.

- It is always a good idea to interview in more than one healthcare facility.

- You will learn as much about the facility from those who work there as you will from the individuals that interview you.

- Your first job sets the stage for the rest of your healthcare career.

- Be sure you determine what type of orientation and specialty education programs are available for new graduate healthcare workers.

- Ask specific questions about how long you will orient, if you will be assigned a preceptor, and when you will be "turned loose" to care for patients on your own.

- If you are not in an orientation program that is at least a month long (including general orientation days), you will not be adequately prepared to function as a healthcare professional.

- Some facilities are beginning to offer RN Residencies for new grads.

- You will need a comprehensive immersion program that is designed to transition newly graduated healthcare workers from a student to a safe, competent professional

- You definitely want to work at a facility with a formal orientation program.

- Insist on formal orientation and an individual preceptor before you accept a new grad position in any healthcare specialty.

Having a Life and a Career: Achieving Life Balance

- Healthcare is a stressful profession, so you need some self care strategies to make the most of your life and your healthcare role.

- When you start a new job, remember you do not have to know everything.

- Even experienced staff start out as a novice when they go into a new role.

- It is okay to not know things. You are not expected to know everything.

- Employers do expect healthcare workers to deliver safe and competent care to patients..

- Ask for help *before* you are drowning or if you are not sure what to do.

- You are responsible for telling your supervisor if you are not trained or have never performed a specific skill that you are asked to do as a new healthcare worker.

- Policies and procedures are created as safeguards to protect patients.

- It is important to know where to find the information you need.

- Find a staff member you can trust to be your mentor or coach.

- Common courtesy and graciousness are as important as your clinical skills for success

- Don't let other staff take advantage of you.

- Consider journaling your ideas, problems, solutions and strategies

- You cannot care for others effectively without caring for yourself first.

Discussion Questions:

1. Explain why a formal orientation program is so important to your first year of success.

2. Identify ways to balance your life and work.

3. Discuss why mentors and/or coaches are so important.

4. Describe in detail the licensure/certification process for your particular specialty.

Case Studies:

1. Candy is a new radiology technologist. She has applied at the facility in her community. They promise her an orientation, a "buddy" and a reasonable salary. What questions should she ask about this offer? Why? What is missing from the offer?

2. Mary is a new grad RN. She started on a medical-surgical floor following graduation. She attended hospital general orientation, and an additional week of clinical orientation. She has a resource RN. Mary is frightened, exhausted, and wants to quit. What would you tell her? Why?

CAREER DEVELOPMENT

Instructor Guide
Chapter 3

CHAPTER 3. CAREER DEVELOPMENT

Chapter Objectives:

1. Define career development and explain why it is important.

2. Discuss and identify the components of career development.

3. Explain the components of the Turner Career Development model ©.

4. List 5 traits of an indispensable healthcare worker.

5. List 2 methods to improve your career

6. Explain the different types of recruiters and which is most useful to your career choice.

Key terms

Career development
Career development model
Indispensable
Career plan
Recruiter

Career enhancement
Career self-assessment
Interview

Key concepts: Career Development

1. Career development means taking total responsibility for your career and your life.

2. Career success requires careful planning and analysis.

3. Every job and role you take allows you to gather more experience, skills and competencies and place in your career "toolkit".

4. The more tools you have in your tool kit, the more marketable you are.

5. Treat your career like a business and manage it.

6. There are identifiable traits of Indispensible employees

7. As important as it is to look backward, it is more important to look ahead

8. Create the right career support structure for career management.

9. Remember that simply doing a good job does not guarantee success.

10. As you gain experience as a healthcare professional, you will need to use a career development plan.

11. Assess your career at regular intervals and actively plan your next steps

Turner Career Development Model©

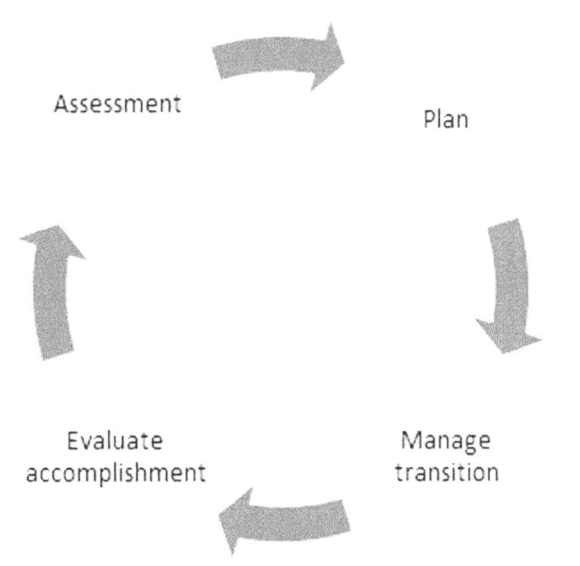

- Career development starts with an assessment of where you are and then determining where you want to be

- When you are living the overwhelming grind of working *towards* your future, you end up thinking that you can always do your wish list someday. Suddenly someday is *NOW.*

- Continue your career management throughout your professional life.

- Pick a date and assess where you are annually.

- Be sure you also consider what you cannot do and what you are not.

- Always keep long term goals in mind

Resumes

- Create a useful resume and

- Create individualized cover letter.

Interviews

- First impressions really do matter.

- Most healthcare interviews now include questions based on a behavioral-based model (case scenarios).

- Don't forget to do your homework. Remember, you are interviewing the facility as much as they are interviewing you.

Working with a Recruiter

- Many hard to find, middle management and senior executive positions are filled by corporate recruiters.

- When contacted by a recruiter you should also ask if he or she is calling about a specific opportunity, a future opportunity, or general career opportunities

- Recruiters want to fill the position and will always look for ways to rule a candidate "in" rather than rule a candidate 'out'.

- Recruiters are like "sellers" agents in real estate □ they work for the company, not for the candidate.

- Most recruiters always assume that candidates are on their "best" behavior during the interview process and that any behavioral "red flags" uncovered during the interviews will only be magnified once you start work.

- Recruiters are a key player in employers' decision making process

Discussion Questions:

1. Discuss pros and cons of career development

2. Identify 3 characteristics/methods to improve your career.

3. Identify 4 components of Turner Career Development model and explain each one.

4. Compare and contrast the types of recruiters and their importance to your career choices.

5. Identify 3 interview questions and your answers to them.

6. List two ways you can enhance your career.

7. Have each student complete self assessment documents. Discuss in small groups to identify trends or issues.

8. Discuss components of a successful interview process.

Case Studies:

1. Alex is a housekeeper in a community hospital. He is married with 5 children. He has worked in this role at the same facility for 20 years. He is interested in a career that will pay more, have less physical demands and will provide a good retirement. How would you assist him?

2. A recruiter calls you to ask if you would be interested in a job as a manager in your area of expertise. It is an existing role in a competing facilities What questions would you ask the recruiter? Why?

CAREER DEVELOPMENT TOOLS

Turner Career Self Assessment Tool©

1. The tasks and components I like most about my present job are:

2. The tasks and components I like least about my present job are:

3. The tasks I excel in at in my present job are:

4. The tasks I struggle with in my present job are:

5. My education goals are:

6. My life long learning goals are:

7. My short term (within one year) goal (s) is (are): By 20___ , I will have:

8. The steps I need to take to achieve this short term goal are:

9. My long term (two to three years) goal (s) is (are): By 20___, I will have:

10. The steps I need to take to achieve this long term goal are:

11. Jobs outside the acute care hospital that interest me are:

12. Areas of cross training or specialization within the hospital that interest me are:

13. The resources I need to achieve my short term and long term goals are:

Turner Healthcare Associates, Inc, ©1994

Turner Career Development Assessment Tool©

1. What are you doing now? Describe your work and role:

2. What do you want and need in a job and role? (list points from the self assessment tool)

3. Gather information about the roles you like: what do you know about these roles? What do you like about them? What else can you find out? Where? When?

4. Target one or two roles to aim for: what is it? Where is it done? Who do you know that you could job shadow in this role?

5. Decide which one role you actually want to do. If you had to make a decision today, what would you choose? Why?

6. List and explain four strategies to achieve the role you chose in the previous question.

7. To implement your strategies you would have to do what? How? When? Where?

8. Is furthering your professional education important to you? Why or why not?

9. If you want to further your professional education, what will you do? When? How?

10. Decide on a method for you to continue your ongoing career development and management. What will the method include? When will you do it?

11. How will you know you are successful at achieving your goal(s)? List your criteria for success.

12. What will you do to reward yourself for your success? When?

Turner Healthcare Associates, Inc. © 1994

 ## Turner Career Planning Process©

1. Where do you want to be in 3-5 years?

2. What do you want and like in a job?

3. Gather information about the roles you like. List them.

4. Target 1-2 roles to aim for. List them.

5. Decide on 1 role to do. List it.

6. Develop 5 strategies to achieve that role (school, certification, job shadow).

7. Implement your 5 strategies, one at a time.

8. Evaluate your outcomes and continue ongoing career management.

Turner Healthcare Associates, Inc, © 1994

Turner Stress Assessment Tool©

For the purposes of this test, stress is defined as a mismatch between the demands placed on you and your ability to meet those demands.

Circle the correct response for you. There are no "right" answers!

1. Do you feel stressed at work?   Yes   No

2. Do you feel more stressed at work now than you did three years ago?   Yes   No

3. Do you feel more stressed at work now than you did one year ago?   Yes   No

4. How stressed to you feel right now?   Not at all   Not much   Fairly   Some   Very

5. If you feel stressed how does this manifest itself? Circle all that apply:

Physically

Headaches   stomach/bowel problems   chest pain   frequent infections
sleep problems   weight loss   weight gain   loss of libido

Psychological

Moodiness/irritability   tiredness   apathy   depression   anxiety

Frustration   indecision   boredom   feeling guilty   poor concentration

Behaviorally

Accident-prone   alcohol abuse   drug abuse   food abuse

Aggressiveness   relationship difficulties   absenteeism

6. How do you feel stress in your personal life affect you at work?

Not at all   a little   quite a bit   a lot

7. How do you feel stress at work affects your personal life?

Not at all   a little   quite a bit   a lot

8. If you feel stressed, what would you say are the major causes of your stress?

Excessive workload   lack of resources   staff-related

Management- related   patient-related   personal difficulties

Changes within profession   job insecurity   job transition/new job

9. How do you cope with stress?

Counseling   support groups   recreational activities relaxation

Stress management techniques   talking with friends/significant other

Regular exercise   alcohol/drugs/nicotine/food   missing work   denial

10. How would you rate your ability to cope with stress?

Poor   Average   Better than average   Very good

11. How many stress-related sick leave/days have you used in the past year?

Turner Indispensable Assessment Tool ©

Are you in a position of being indispensable to your boss or unit? Take this assessment to see how indispensable you are. The more yes answers you have, the more indispensable you are!

1. Are you clinically competent?

2. Do you have general understanding of JCAHO accreditation and requirements?

3. Do you have general understanding of managed care issues that affect your geographic area?

4. Do you have general understanding of budget and cost issues that affect your facility?

5. Are you willing to be a partner with your institution, not just an employee?

6. Do you have decision making skills?

7. Are you self directed, not always expecting to be told what to do?

8. Do you have integrity?

9. Do you have an objective perspective?

10. Do you act like a victim?

11. Do you have a strong work ethic? (not a workaholic)

12. Do you have a high energy level?

13. Do you have effective time management skills?

14. Do you have a strong positive self image?

15. Do you have effective interpersonal skills

16. Are you flexible?

17. Are you excited, not threatened by change?

18. Can you deal with change and get mobilized, even if you are afraid?

19. Are you adaptable?

20. Are you assertive?

21. Are you tenacious?

22. Do you have personal ambition and drive?

23. Are you self-motivated and a self-starter?

GENERAL CAREER SKILLS

Chapter 4 Instructor Guide

CHAPTER 4. GENERAL CAREER SKILLS

Chapter Objectives:

1. Define and explain the importance soft skills.

2. List 4 soft skills that are critical to career success

3. Discuss ways to sell your potential with no career experience.

4. Explain the Parieto principle and why it matters in your career.

5. List 5 examples of effective time management.

6. List the 3 keys to managing time.

7. List 3 things your boss wants you to know.

8. Identify and explain the successful communication sequence.

9. List 3 barriers to effective communication.

Key terms

Soft skills
Communication
Time management
Parieto principle
Self confidence
Organizational skills

Political skills
Vibrating poles
Critical thinking
What your boss wants

Important Job Skills

- In addition to technical and professional skills, employers are also looking for other skills. These other skills are often called "soft skills"

- Soft job skills are just as important as clinical competencies and include:

  - Oral/spoken communication skills

  - Written communication skills

  - Being truthful and having integrity

  - Working effectively with others to accomplish tasks

  - Self-motivation/initiative = Doing things without needing to be told or persuaded

  - Work ethic/dependability = Being thorough and accurate so others can count on you

  - Critical thinking = Challenging things when appropriate and proposing alternatives to consider

  - Risk-taking skills = Taking a considered chance on something new, different or unknown

  - Flexibility/adaptability = Going with the flow and adjusting with unforeseen circumstances

  - Influencing skills = Persuading others to think about or adopt a different point of view

  - Organization skills = Being organized and methodical, especially in work-related situations

  - Problem-solving skills = Analyzing the potential causes of a problem and creating a solution

  - Multicultural skills = Understanding and relating to people who are different from you

  - Computer skills = Using basic word-processing, spreadsheet and presentation software as well as the Internet

  - Academic/learning skills = Learning new things quickly, thoroughly, and being willing to learn continuously

- Making sure that even the little things are done and done correctly

- Teaching/training skills = Showing other people how to do something in a way that allows them to learn quickly and clearly

- Guiding and supporting others in order to accomplish something

- Relating with other people and communicating with them in everyday interactions

- Handling the stress that accompanies deadlines and other limitations or constraints

- Asking questions in order to learn or clarify something

- Having the imagination to come up with new or out-of–the-box ideas

- Quantitative skills = Compiling and using numbers to study an issue or answer a question

- Research skills = Gathering information to answer questions.

- Time management skills = Using your time wisely and consistently staying on schedule and meeting deadlines. (Vought,2005)

Selling Yourself with no Experience

- One of the biggest challenges in the work place is selling your self without having experience.

- Must sell job performance potential, and that's what you need to highlight

- A positive, upbeat, eager, self-confident attitude is critical (not arrogance

- Demonstrate your willingness to take an entry-level position.

- The quicker you can learn the business of your specialty as well as healthcare, the quicker you can expect to move up within the organization.

- Demonstrate your desire to learn.

- Have reasonable salary expectations.

- Every new employee brings a different set of skills, training, experience and ability to the job.

- When employers are asked to rank the three most important skills they look for in new

- Don't rely on just your degree.

- A degree won't get you a job– it will just open the door.

- All you really can expect is the chance to prove what you can do.

What your boss wants you to know

- There are certain basic social and political skills that are required in virtually every job.

- These are the things your boss wishes you knew even if s/he hasn't told you.

- If you have a boss that displays behaviors that you see are perceived as unacceptable by fellow employees or administrators, take note of that as well.

- You can always learn what *not* to do at the same time you are learning what to do well.

- Many healthcare facilities are extremely dysfunctional, so we can't change anything. As we continue to try and control whatever is dysfunctional, the more frustrated we get, and still nothing changes.

- A healthcare organization is the equivalent of a vibrating pole. The temptation is to hang on to the pole to make it stop vibrating. In reality, that makes both you and the pole vibrate. The answer is to let go of the pole.

Time Management

- Even if you are not a manager, everyone can use ideas and tools to better manage time.

- Time management is not about the amount of time we have. It is how we utilize the time that is available to us.

- Time is our most valuable resource.

- Time has special characteristics.

- There are many reasons why people don't manage their work time well.

- Barriers and excuses keep you from managing your time effectively.

- `You must develop job objectives and priorities

- Analyze how you use your time

- Have a results-oriented plan (outcomes-based)

- Organize for achievement

- Peter Drucker, believes that the key to effectiveness is to know where our time should be spent for the results we want.

- The Pareto Principle (80/20) provides that 80% of our results come from 20% of what we do.

- There are many things that are time wasters.

- You can form new habits for each time waster and gain time.

- Real time management is self management.

- Good time managers are good at controlling their responses to events they can't control.

- Set priorities so that what is important is what is accomplished.

- Delegation is an effective time management strategy

Evaluate your Communication Styles— It Does Affect your Career

- Communication is an active process, not a static one.

- Communication is the sending and receiving of information, feelings and attitudes, both verbally and non-verbally, that produces a response (2012).

- Effective communication occurs between two persons when the receiver interprets the sender's message the same way that the sender intended it.

- A successful communication sequence looks like this:

Sender☐ Meaning☐ Message☐ Symbols☐ Meaning☐ Receiver (Turner, 1999)

- The same factors that create effective communication can also be barriers to effective communications.

- There are other barriers to effective communication include

- Healthcare staff can use strategies to improve communication and become successful at communication in the workplace.

- During stressful times, effective communication becomes critical.

- Timing of communication is crucial.

- Non-verbal communication is the most important aspect of communication and often the most ignored.

- Focus on issues and behaviors, not people.

- Listening is a critical element of the communication process.

Discussion Questions:

1. Discuss and explain the importance soft skills.

2. Identify 4 soft skills that are critical to career success and why.

3. Discuss ways to sell your potential with no career experience.

4. Explain the Parieto principle and why it matters in your career.

5. Discuss and identify effective time management skills.

6. Discuss the keys to managing time and how to use them.

7. Discuss and explain the concept of "things your boss wants you to know". List examples.

8. Discuss and explain the successful communication sequence.

9. Discuss barriers to effective communication, and why they happen.

Case Studies:

1. Eileen is new in her role as CEO of a hospital non-profit foundation (fund raising arm). Her role is to manage existing donations as well as obtain more monies. She is also in charge of the operations of a six person department. She reports to the facility CEO and sits on the management council. What skills are most important in her role? Why?

2. Rita is an Emergency Department (ED) nurse who applied for a new role as Pre-Hospital Care coordinator. It is a promotion within the ED. When she was not selected, she wrote a letter to the Department manager, the VP of Patient Care, the Chief of the Medical Staff and the hospital CEO. Why do you think she did this? Was this appropriate? Why or why not? What could she have done differently?

SUPERVISION AND MANAGEMENT OF WORKERS

*Chapter 5
Instructor Guide*

CHAPTER 5. SUPERVISION AND MANAGEMENT

Chapter Objectives:

1. Define the role of a supervisor

2. Explain the difference between authoritarian and participative management styles.

3. Discuss the concept of discipline.

4. List 6 unforgivable supervisory mistakes.

5. Explain the different management theories including theory X,Y,Z,C,T

6. Identify 6 differences between managers and leaders.

7. Explain the process of decision making

8. Explain the process of problem solving

Key terms

Supervision	Management techniques	Delegation
Power	Influence	
Management	Discipline	
Leadership	Decision making	
Problem solving	Management theories	

Key Concepts: Supervising the work of others

- A supervisor, more than anything else, is a leader.

- The supervisor accomplishes tasks through other people so that the organization's goals can be achieved.

- Some supervisors appear to have natural leadership ability, but most supervisors have had to develop their skills through experience and training.

- There are different leadership styles

- To be effective, supervisors must have priorities on what to do.

- As a supervisor, one of the most important tasks is that of teaching and training.

- Supervisors are also responsible for safety on the unit.

- The most difficult responsibility of a supervisor is discipline

- A positive attitude as a supervisor affects productivity

- Six Unforgivable Supervisory Mistakes

  - Treating individuals unequally because of sex, culture, age, disability, etc.

  - Not keeping your word.

  - Blowing hot and cold.

  - Failure to follow basic company/facility policies and procedures.

  - Losing your cool in front of staff.

  - Engaging in a personal relationship with someone you supervise.

Successful/unsuccessful supervisory traits

Successful supervisors	Unsuccessful supervisors
Remain positive under stress	Permit problems to get to them
Take time to teach what they know	Rush instructions to staff, then fail to follow-up
Build/maintain rewarding relationships with subordinates	Insensitive to subordinates needs
Learn to set reasonable and consistent lines of authority	Not interested in learning supervisory skills
Learn to delegate	Fail to understand that it isn't what a supervisor can do, but what they can get others to accomplish
Establish standards of high quality and set good examples	Let their status go to their head
Work hard to become good communicators	Continue to offer one way communication
Build team efforts to achieve high productivity	Become too authoritarian or too lax

Effective supervision includes:

- Being organized so you have more time for goal setting and dealing with subordinates

- Delegate effectively

- Communicate effectively

- Discipline appropriately

Supervisors that Delegate effectively:

- Explain importance of job

38

- Explain end results and let the employee determine how the task will e completed

- Clearly define the employee's authority and/or parameters that the employee has when completing the task

- Agree on a deadline and time frame with the employee

- Ask for feedback to ensure the employee completely understands the tasks and your expectations

- Provide controls to ensure the employee is on the right track. Follow-up and check on the employee's progress on the task.

Supervisors that communicate effectively:

- Plan for the communication with the employee. Schedule a time and plan what you want to say.

- Be honest, candid, specific and factual. Provide examples

- Open up communication with open ended questions. Remember to listen, as it needs to be two way communication

- Ask for feedback. Ensure that you and the employee have a shared understanding of the goal. Everyone has the need to feel important enough to be asked for their views.

Supervisors that discipline appropriately:

- Give facts and figures unemotionally

- Help the employee understand why s/he is being disciplined, and define the problem.

- Get agreement that a problem exists

- Look for solutions to resolve the performance problem/conduct

What skills are required in a Charge Role?

- Most healthcare facilities have someone in charge of each unit or shift.

- Whatever the title, the role includes direct accountability for one unit on one shift.

- This is the first step in becoming a supervisor and usually a step before becoming a manager.

- Outstanding charge personnel are easy to spot and have specific characteristics

- Lack of communication by healthcare managers is a key reason for conflict with staff members

- The charge personnel become a crucial conduit for the healthcare manager with staff on a unit.

- Mentoring and support for new charge personnel, as well as resources and training are crucial to their success.

- Charge personnel need to be selected on their ability to supervise the work of others, not just because they are good clinicians.

- Being a manager is the most challenging role in healthcare

- There are key experience, attributes and characteristics of charge personnel in today's healthcare industry

- There are several leadership theories that have been outlined in the business world over the past several decades. In a nutshell these are:

Leadership Theory	Driving thought
Theory X	No one really wants to work
Theory Y	Individuals really want to make a contribution
Theory Z	People work best in teams
Theory C	If you satisfy the customer, you will have a future
Transformational leadership theory	Visionary, risk taker, confidence builder, and change artist

There are difference between managers and leaders:

Managers	Leaders
Do things right	Do the right things
Solve problems	Avoid problems
Follow direction	Obtain results
Manage productivity	Increase profits
Are efficient	Are effective
Maintain compliance	Improve the system
Control	Influence
Work in hierarchy	Work in network
Make plans	Enhance learning
Create transaction	Create transformation
Administers	Innovates
Copies	Starts from original
Maintains	Develops
Focuses on systems and structure	Focuses on people
Relies on control	Inspires trust
Uses short range viewpoint	Uses long range perspective
Keeps eyes on bottom line	Has eyes on the horizon
Asks how and when	Asks what and why
Accepts the status quo	Challenges status quo
Classic good soldier	Own individual person

- Leaders for professional staff are like yeast is to bread or fuel is to a rocket.

- Supervisory skills are crucial

Charge personnel core competencies include:

- Problem solving

- Management

- Influence

- Social and communication skills

- Achievement

- Self-management

- Keeps external focus

- Promotes vision and values for the future

- Promotes continual quality and process improvement

- Acts as a change agent

- Values people

- Demonstrates skills of management especially under circumstances of uncertainty or conflict

- Decentralizes information and authority

- Pursues self development

Should You Be A Healthcare Manager?

- Managers are paid to make tough decisions.

- What is required to do the job well is not just being in control, but gaining the support and commitment of subordinates, peers and higher-ups as collaborators.

- Formal authority can often effect changes in behavior, but for commitment or changes in attitude, managers have to share their power.

- Empowerment means sharing the potential to influence others.

- Sharing power with others actually increases a manager's influence.

- When a manager creates allies, s/he enhances her/his influence as well as the ability to get the job done.

- Trust will drive your source of power.

- Mutual trust will allow you to build influence.

- Trust is a function of how an individual perceives a manager in three areas. These area are competence (does s/he know the right thing to do?), character (does s/he want to do the right thing?) and influence (can s/he get it done?).

- To work, networks have to be mutually beneficial.

- Treating people fairly is to treat them differently – based on what *they* need.

Responsibilities of managers in leadership roles

Be the source of a vision
Establish and maintain trust
Serve as a political conduit
Serve as ethical standard bearer for the unit/department
Make decisions
Make effective and appropriate judgments
Expand awareness of staff
Become a spark
Build a framework for effective communication
Adopt a constant planning perspective and attitude

- Being a manager can be one of the most rewarding career moves a healthcare worker can make.

- Being a manager involves being a leader, as well as supervising the work of others.

- Expanding your job-related education is an effective way to move ahead.

- The ability to motivate others and oversee their work is critical in most healthcare roles

- Making decisions and delegation are key functions of managers.

- Managers must be able to operate independently and be self-directed.

- The ability to listen, explain clearly and give precise directions is crucial.

- Don't fall into the common trap of assuming people will know how to act if you are their manager.

- one of the real tests of your skills as a manager is the effect you have on the majority of people who don't know what you want intuitively.

- Decide what you want your staff to know.

- Reward good work and that behavior will happen more often

- Groups of people and team members will invariably experience conflict.

- Be sure you share information.

- It takes time for new managers to learn how to be effective.

Risks of being a manager	Rewards of being a manager
Inability to be positive 100% of time	Empowerment
Increased stress	Increased self confidence
Lack of security	Expanding horizons
Feel "caught in the middle"	Personal growth
Crises orientated basis of function	Satisfaction from helping others grow
Changing relationships	Building professionalism/pride
Failure	Success
"Doesn't feel fun anymore"	Feel passionate and excited about work

- Facilities cannot ignore the effect that leadership style has on retention.

- Toxic healthcare executives and middle managers can sabotage retention efforts

- A positive leadership style is a cornerstone of success as well as a key retention strategy.

- Never forget what it's like to be in the trenches.

- Graciousness and common courtesy go a long way.

- Build trust.

- Relationship management matters.

- Being a good manager is not being popular.

- Never ask someone to do something you wouldn't do yourself.

- If you ask staff members their opinions, be prepared to do something with the answers.

- Manage by walking around.

- Delegate; then get out of the way.

- Embrace and manage change.

- Be a risk taker.

- Strive to become a leader, not just a manager

- Build bridges not kingdoms.

- Being a good manager means empowerment.

- Communicate often and tell the truth

- Use the 24 hour rule

- Remember that people are like popcorn:

- Let go of vibrating poles:

- Make sure you fight over only silver bullets:

- Remember that the patient is what matters the most:

Old way of managing (authoritarian)	New way of managing (participative)
Rigidly defined individual responsibilities	Flexible definition of responsibilities of team members via discussion and consensus
Fosters competition between individuals	Fosters cooperation and teamwork among members
Assumes that staff are passive, lack ambition and need controlling	Assumes that staff have motivation and readiness to direct behavior toward organizational goals
Management is to direct, control and motivate others	Arrange organizational conditions and operations so staff can achieve their on goals best by directing efforts toward organizational objectives
Quality is fine the way it is	Quality can and must improve
Checking data/reports ensures quality	Analysis and improving processes ensures quality
People cause defects and poor quality	Processes and systems cause defects and poor quality
Intuition and technology will solve problems	Collecting data and acting with knowledge will solve problems
Quality costs money	Quality saves money
Customers are problems	Customers are partners
Suppliers/vendors are problems	Suppliers/vendors are partners
We don't have time for quality and customer service	We don't have time not to have quality and customer service

Managing an Effective Team

- The key to success as a supervisor or manager is the relationship between you and your work group.

- Organizations utilize the concept of synergy that teamwork can accomplish much more than its individual members can do by working alone.

- Calling a group a team doesn't make it a team.

- Teamwork is accomplished by making sure that cooperative behavior is positively reinforced.

- The most effective healthcare work environment is one when people know when to work alone and when to ask for help.

- There are several essential elements that differentiate a team from a group of people. Within teams:

  - The group members must have shared goals or a reason for working together

  - The group members must be interdependent on each others' experience, abilities and commitment in order to achieve mutual goals

  - The group members must be committed to the idea that working together leads to more effective decisions than working alone

  - The group must be accountable as a functioning unit within a larger organizational context e.g. a hospital (Reilly,1974)

  - Quality care and efficient service means working together

  - An effective team member has the following characteristics:

    - Understands and is committed to team goals

    - Is friendly, concerned and interested in others

    - Acknowledges and confronts conflict openly

- Listens to others with understanding

- Includes others in the decision making process

- Recognizes and respects individual differences

- Contributes ideas and solutions

- Values and respects others' ideas and contributions

- Recognizes and rewards team efforts

- Encourages and appreciates feedback about team performance

- An effective team is one that can solve its own problems, and the ability to solve problems is predicated on an ability to identify and remove obstacles that deflect energy from those problems.

- As a team leader you can help ensure the effectiveness of your team by helping your team members recognize their strengths and abilities.

- Treat your team members as well as you want them to treat patients.

- Understanding your group member dynamics will make you a more effective supervisor.

- The supervisor is an important part of the total team system. Highly effective work groups see their supervisors as:

  - Supportive, friendly and helpful

  - Having confidence in their ability and integrity

  - Having high performance expectations

  - Providing necessary training and coaching

  - Viewing errors as learning opportunities rather than chances to criticize

Self interested individuals destroy teamwork success.

The supervisor's attitude and involvement patterns tend to be mirrored in the behavior of the group members.

Supervisors need to manage team members more as a coach than a boss. This means that staff needs to understand in behavioral terms what they are do to. You must clarify what group members are to do in a coaching way:

Supervisory behaviors	Coaching behaviors
Hand out assignments	Develop a positive reinforcement plan
Tell people how to do a job	Give performance feedback
Keep people on task	Share information
Find and punish poor performance	Mediate reinforcement between team members
Protect organization information	Deliver positive reinforcement for decision making, creative solutions, cooperation and initiative.

- The best way to empower team members is gradually and systematically.

- Once you have an effective team, everyone's job will be easier

Each team member and discipline must function within their scope of practice.

- Standards of practice and role-based competencies drive different roles, functions and tasks.

- Accountability is also a function of team work.

- Commitment is part of being a team.

- Newly constructed teams go through several stages before they work well together. Tuckman lists four stages of team development.

These stages are:

- Forming: getting started; getting to know each other, not sure what to do

- Storming: going in circles, having trouble working together; focused on end goal instead of process of getting work done.

- Norming: getting on course, now know each other; identify goal and work together

- Performing: work at full speed ahead; working together to achieve goal; use feedback to make changes and look for ways to improve

Some teams are dysfunctional and never get out of the storming phase.

Committees and unit teams that are effectively have successfully worked through all four stages one size coaching DOES NOT fit all

> Placing emphasis on problem solving, not blaming

> Recognizing obstacles and change are facts of life for teams

> Teams require effective personal communication:

> Delegation to other team members:

> When working with a team, listening is more important than talking

Effective Delegation

- No matter how effective you are as a supervisor, there is a limit to the capacity you can accomplish as a working supervisor.

- Successful supervisors know when and what to delegate.

- Delegation is the assignment of authority for the completion of tasks to others.

- One of the major concepts of delegation is to provide your subordinates with the necessary information and authority to complete the tasks assigned, but you retain the responsibility for the final achievement of the goals or outcome.

- As you increase the responsibilities of your subordinates, you expand your own ability to manage more effectively

- Many supervisors believe that delegating means assigning parts of their work to someone else that they don't want to do. This is not delegating. It is dumping.

- There are certain tasks you cannot delegate to others as a supervisor.

- You must also assess how much authority you can delegate to others based on the tasks assigned

- Delegating a portion of your authority to a subordinate does not relieve you of your responsibility to your boss and the organization to ensure these duties are properly completed.

- you must also establish controls for the type of work assigned.

- Delegation has several steps to ensure delegation with effective results.

- Once an assignment is completed, be sure to give your subordinate credit for a job well done.

- You take responsibility if the assignment was less than successful.

Delegation Dos and Don'ts

DO	DON'T
Encourage free flow of information to subordinates	Hoard information
Focus on results	Emphasize methods
Delegate through dialogue	Do all the talking yourself
Fix firm deadlines	Leave timeframes unclear or uncertain
Make sure the person has all the necessary resources	Half delegate by giving assignments without the needed tools and information
Delegate the entire task to one person	Delegate half the task
Give advice without interfering	Fail to point out pitfalls

Build controls into the process of delegating	Impose controls as an afterthought
Back up those delegated to in legitimate disputes	Leave persons to fight their own battles on your behalf
Give the delegate full credit for his/her accomplishments	Hog the glory or look for a scapegoat

Turner Delegation Self Assessment Checklist©

Check all that apply:

1. Your workload has prevented you from taking regular vacations.

2. You feel overworked frequently.

3. You leave jobs unfinished.

4. You take work home most nights and weekends.

5. It always seems you have more work than your subordinates.

6. Planning is a low priority task for you.

7. You have no time for outside activities.

8. In the past week, you have engaged in detail work that isn't your job.

9. You do your subordinates' work for them frequently.

10. Crises and problems are more common in your job than opportunities.

11. Often you haven't had time to fully explain a task to your subordinate.

12. You frequently have problems meeting your boss's deadlines.

13. You like to keep your hands in your old job.

14. You are a perfectionist– and proud of it!

15. You wish you had more time in your personal life.

16. You can't think of your top three current work goals.

17. You believe in giving subordinates only the information they need to do their specific jobs.

18. You rarely elicit the opinions of your subordinates about anything.

19. In your opinion, your subordinates are not to be trusted with too much information.

20. It is hard for you to accept ideas offered by someone else.

21. You get the feeling that sometimes your subordinates are trying to undermine you.

22. You believe your subordinates are coasting.

23. Your subordinates' think how something is done is more important than what is achieved.

24. Your staff refuses to make any decisions without consulting you first.

25. Your staff comes to you for advice on their work more than necessary.

26. Your staff exceeds their authority regularly.

27. Your staff acts according to the literal rather than the spirit of an assignment.

28. Sometimes, your staff consults with you after the fact about significant actions.

29. None of your staff could fill in for you if you got run over by a bus.

30. Your staff turns work assignments back to you and you accept them.

31. Your staff wouldn't work at all if you weren't there to push them to do tasks.

32. Your staff has skills essentially unchanged from a year ago.

33. Staff rarely comes to you with new ideas or new ways of doing their jobs.

Evaluating and Critiquing Performance

- Evaluating performance is a process that happens over time.

- A performance evaluation is an opportunity to assess the demonstrated performance of team members and staff over a period of time.

- The evaluation communicates the assessment and expectations for the future. The two most frequently mentioned responses to studies on what is most important to people about their work were communication and recognition.

- Not providing information makes staff members think you are deliberately keeping bad news from them.

- Staff expects communication and recognition from their direct supervisor.

- An evaluation gives a supervisor the chance to accurately communicate how a staff member is performing their job, restate expectations and set new goals

- Performance evaluations give the supervisor an opportunity to recognize staff performance and praise strengths as well as identify areas to improve.

- Getting a performance evaluation should mean no surprises for the staff member.

- Clear communication is a large part of the performance evaluation process.

- It is critical to concentrate on job performance–not the staff member's personality–when making this assessment.

Timely

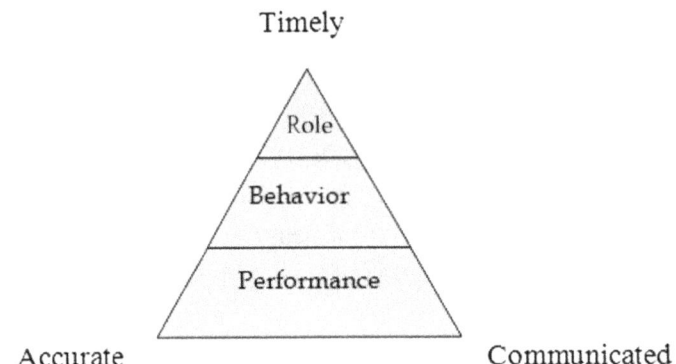

Accurate   Communicated

- Performance evaluations can be thought of as a triangle. It must be accurate, communicated and timely.

- When completing a performance evaluation, be on time with completion of the evaluation.

- Consider the staff members performance for the entire time period. Do not base your assessment on only the most recent weeks or months. Use examples of both positive and negative performance.

- Schedule time to meet with the employee.

- Encourage the staff member to participate with input and comments

- Avoid confrontation and argument with the employee.

- Listen with objectivity and stress performance, not personality or attitude.

- Set new goals, considering progress, growth, future, and employee development.

- Establish a plan and time table to meet those objectives with the employee

- Employees deserve to know the consequences of not performing to expectations.

- Say "thank you" for your associate's participation in the meeting and their contribution for the year.

- There are specific ways to describe both positive and negative employee behaviors in a written performance evaluation.

Positive Behaviors	Negative Behaviors
Methodical	Needs many explanations
Generates enthusiasm	Perfectionist
Willing to accept difficult assignments	Slow to get things done; resists difficult materials
Pays attention to deadlines	Overreacts to criticism
Avoids risks	Tends to day dream
Gets tasks done	Unprepared
Accountable for own work	Shifts blame to others
Sets and completes goals	Disorganized
Sensitive when showing disapproval	Unfriendly to patients; inefficient
Willing to help others succeed	Does not check work before submission
Obtains needed information	Resists changes
Shares information with others	Disrupts meetings
Maintains high standards	Takes shortcuts
Flexible	Sensitive to criticism
Becomes adaptable to those in authority	Resist participation in team; displays superior attitude
Gives recognition to others	Overuses enthusiasm
Takes on challenges	Displays frustration
Works calmly in unpredictable environment	Under pressure becomes soft and persuadable
Good organizer	Easily intimidated
Good listener; team player	Fails to communicate information, directions, feelings
Innovative	Shows little imagination
Makes good decisions quickly	Makes decisions too fast
Diplomatic with people	Abrupt with others

Providing Discipline to staff members

- Formal progressive discipline is a last resort for sharing expectations with employees.

- If employee performance is a problem, then numerous discussions and clarification of performance expectations should take place before the disciplinary process begins.

- Progressive discipline is used to correct a deficiency in conduct, performance, or a violation of policy in an effort to meet established standards of job performance to preserve employment, and to encourage staff to behave sensibly and safely at work.

- Progressive discipline is continually forward focused instruction and education process.

- Staff needs to hear what they are doing right as well as feedback on problematic personnel issues.

- Staff expects just and equal treatment in which the discipline is in line with the performance problem or misconduct.

- If the supervisor is a good leader, shows a sincere interest in staff and makes work enjoyable, the staff is far less likely to break rules or cause problems

- If you are a supervisor and expected to administer progressive discipline, become familiar with the policy *before* you need to implement it.

- There are instances where termination is immediate for gross misconduct

- One of the most important aspects of the disciplinary process is to determine whether it is truly called for.

- A complete and impartial investigation into the situation must be conducted before discipline is issued.

- If you must conduct a disciplinary meeting with an employee, schedule it after the investigation is completed.

- Make an appointment, and ensure complete privacy.

- It is much easier to coach and supervise employees instead of disciplining them.

- Discipline should be used as a corrective action.

Decision making

- Katz identified three essential management skill sets: technical, human and conceptual. (Robbins)

- Technical skills are those that encompass the ability to apply specialized knowledge or expertise.

- Human skills are those that demonstrate ability to work with, understand and motivate other people, both individually and in groups.

- A key concept that affects managers' abilities to get things done is their ability to manage problem solving and make decisions.

- Problem solving and decision making are based on perception.

- People don't *see* reality. They *interpret* what they see and call it reality.

- Numerous factors that influence perception. Attitudes, motives, interests, experience and expectations all affect how people view a situation.

- There is a link between perception and decision making.

- Decision making occurs as a reaction to a problem

- Every decision requires interpretation and evaluation of information.

- The Optimizing Decision Making Model describes how individuals should behave in order to maximize an outcome. (Robbins) There are six steps to this process.

- Rationality means choices that are consistent, objective, logical and value maximizing. Rational decision making implies that the decision maker can be fully objective and logical with a clear goal.(Robbins)

- Decision making is not just an analysis of facts. There is an element of "gut feel" to the process

Steps in Optimizing Decision Making

1. Ascertain the need for a decision

2. Identify the decision criteria

3. Allocate weights to the criteria

4. Develop alternatives

5. Evaluate alternatives

6. Select the best alternative

Problem Solving

- Problem solving requires good decision making.

- Problem solving is a process. Robbins identifies a nine step process of problem solving

- The apparent problem is what you think caused the issue. The root problem is what actually went wrong.

- Problem solving teams try to bring all stakeholders together.

- It is important to collect and analyze data with the idea of resolving the issue.

- There are organizations that continually collect data, but rarely do anything with the information.

- Be sure to include everyone who can help resolve a problem.

- Brainstorming is the time for listing all ideas without judgment or commentary.

- Faulty implementation of a plan can make a good decision ineffective.

- Effective implementation of a plan can make a debatable choice successful.

- Solving the root problem is only half of the solution. Implementation of a plan is what will complete the cycle.

- When teams work together on problem solving, they often get stuck in terms of their ability to move through a problem to the solution.

- Many times the "stuckness" is caused by conflict.

Symptoms of a "Stuck" Team

- Loss of energy
- Helplessness/victimization
- Lack of purpose/identity
- Dishonesty and lack of candor
- Cynicism and mistrust
- Personal attacks made behind team members' backs
- Finger pointing
- When managing the conflict in a team, remember that problem solving efforts must include members from conflicting groups.
- The most helpful strategy for conflict resolution involves refocusing team members on the shared group goal(s).
- Keep the focus is on patient outcomes
- Have the team re-visit the goals and expected outcomes of care on a regular basis to ensure that the quality improvement process is inherent in daily practice.
- Team conflict can also be triggered by transition and change.
- Change makes many people uncomfortable.
- Change involves letting go of old practices and expectations, but can also mean doing your job more effectively.
- Change often causes fear, grief and loss.
- People are like popcorn and "pop" (adapt) to change and new ideas at different times.
- Care management is critical to achieve positive patient outcomes and a perfect fit for both the patient and the team approach.
- Keep the perspective of the "total patient"; not just "tasks".
- Bedside care management improves utilization of resources, job satisfaction and decreases patient length of stay.

Discussion Questions:

1. Define the role of a supervisor, identifying important traits and tasks.

2. Explain the difference between authoritarian and participative management styles, how they differ in the workplace, including results with both styles.

3. Discuss the concept of discipline as a supervisor.

4. List 6 unforgivable supervisory mistakes.

5. Explain the different management theories including theory X,Y,Z,C,T, comparing and contrasting each style in the healthcare workplace.

6. Identify 6 differences between managers and leaders and explain why you chose them.

7. Explain the process of decision making, both positive and negative methods,

8. Explain the process of problem solving, both positive and negative methods.

9. Discuss the meanings of each component in this essay about leadership:

PORTRAIT OF A LEADER

- Persistence. Not insistence. A strong leader hangs on a little longer, works a little harder.

- Imagination. S/he harnesses imagination to practical plans that produce results.

- Vision. The present is just the beginning. A good leader is impressed with the possibilities of the future.

- Sincerity. A good leader can be trusted.

- Integrity. A good leader has principles and lives by them.

- Poise. A good leader is not overbearing, but friendly and assured.

- Thoughtfulness. S/he is considerate and aware.

- Common Sense. A good leader has good judgment based on reason

- Altruism. A good leader lives by the Golden Rule.

- Initiative. S/he gets things started now!

Author unknown

Role play/Interview questions. These can also be used for other chapters of the Instructor Guide, or used for additional essay questions.

Case Study/Role Play:

Opening statement: you have achieved a position of leadership in our healthcare community. Could you tell me a bit about your background and the role you are in today?

1. How would you describe a leader?

2. What are important qualities or characteristics of a leader?

3. Explain your personal philosophy of leadership.

4. What learning experiences have had the most influence on your personal development as a leader?

5. How do you see leadership evolving in healthcare today?

6. What are the most challenging issues in your current positions? Why?

7. As a leader/manager in your career, have you had a mentor? If so, how did this impact your leadership style. If not, why did you not use a mentor and how did that affect your style?

8. What advice would you give someone aspiring to a leadership position?

HEALTHCARE ROLES

Chapter 6
Instructor Guide

CHAPTER 6: HEALTHCARE ROLES

Chapter Objectives:

1. Identify 5 non-clinical roles available in hospitals, and the additional education required, if any, for each role.

2. List 3 non-clinical roles outside hospitals.

3. Explain concept of advanced practice nursing and give examples of roles.

4. Identify 3 advanced practice roles for other healthcare specialties and explain each.

Key terms

Non clinical role

Healthcare executive roles

Advanced practice role

Special focused roles

Community based roles

Occupational Outlook Handbook

Key Concepts

There are Non clinical roles in hospitals:

- Patient/Staff Educators

- Quality Improvement

- Risk Managers

- Case Managers

- Chart Auditors

- Patient Advocates

- Preceptors

- Clinical Information System Consultants

- Clinical Informatics Specialists

Roles in the Community:

- Correctional Healthcare workers

- Forensic Healthcare workers

- Holistic Healthcare workers

- Parish Healthcare workers

- Legal Healthcare Consulting

- Healthcare Consultant

- Medical Office Manager

- Research Healthcare worker

- Case Managers

- Telemedicine Healthcare workers

- Cruise Ship Healthcare workers

- Pharmaceutical, Medical Equipment and Supply Educators

- School Healthcare workers

- Occupational/environmental Healthcare workers

- Broadcast Journalists

- Architectural Building Design/Construction Management

- Healthcare Educators and Faculty

Advanced Practice Roles

- Nurse Practitioners

- Certified Registered Nurse Anesthetists

- Certified Nurse Midwives

- Clinical Nurse Specialists

- Chief Healthcare Executives

- Dental lab technician

- Orthotics/Prosthetics

- Physicians Assistant

- Surgical Assistant/First Assistant

Additional roles and job information can be found within 2010-11 edition of the *Occupational Outlook Handbook* include additional roles such as:

Audiologists

Cardiovascular technologists and technicians

Chiropractors

Clinical laboratory technologists and technicians

Dental assistants

Dental hygienists

Dentists

Diagnostic medical sonographers

Dietitians and nutritionists

Emergency medical technicians and paramedics

Home health aides and personal and home care aides

Licensed practical and licensed vocational nurses

Medical and health services managers

Medical assistants

Medical, dental, and ophthalmic laboratory technicians

Medical records and health information technicians

Medical transcriptionists

Nuclear medicine technologists

Nursing and psychiatric aides

Occupational therapist assistants and aides

Occupational therapists

Opticians, dispensing

Optometrists

Pharmacists

Pharmacy technicians and aides

Physical therapist assistants and aides

Physical therapists

Physician assistants

Physicians and surgeons

Podiatrists

Psychologists

Radiation therapists

Receptionists and information clerks

Recreational therapists

Registered nurses

Respiratory therapists

Respiratory therapy technicians

Social and human service assistants

Speech-language pathologists

Surgical technologists

Discussion Questions:

1. Identify non-clinical roles available in hospitals, and the additional education for each role. What is most practical for your specialty? Why?

2. List 3 non-clinical roles outside hospitals.

3. Explain concept of advanced practice nursing and give examples of roles.

4. Identify 3 advanced practice roles for other healthcare specialties and explain each.

5. Choose 4 additional healthcare roles listed in the Job Outlook Handbook and explain:

    a. Role

    b. Work location

    c. Education/experience required

    d. Potential for job opportunities

Case Studies:

1. Laura is an experienced aerobics and cardio workout instructor. She currently works as an instructor for a national gym chain. She is interested in pursuing a career in healthcare. She has a general studies AA degree from a local community college. She is in a relationship, with 2 kids. What would you suggest to her for healthcare career options?

2. Drew is a recent high school graduate, 2010. He has entered nursing school and failed the second semester at a community college. He still wants to work in healthcare. What kind of roles would you recommend? He is unmarried and needs to work while in school.

ENCOURAGING OTHERS:
MENTORING, COACHING, AND PRECEPTING

Chapter 7
Instructor Guide

CHAPTER 7. ENCOURAGING OTHERS: MENTORING, COACHING, AND PRECEPTING

Chapter Objectives:

1. Define and explain mentoring.

2. Define and explain coaching and why it is necessary.

3. Compare and contrast the differences between coaching and mentoring.

4. Explain the role of preceptor and why it is important to new healthcare workers.

Key terms

Coaching   Mentoring
Preceptor

Effective Mentoring

- Coaches and mentors can help individuals successfully navigate multiple challenges, changes and demands.

- The need for coaching and mentoring has never been more apparent for leaders at

- There is a difference between mentoring and precepting.

- Healthcare professionals interested in mentoring usually like sharing what they know.

- They are willing to share their own good and bad experiences,

- "Good judgment comes from experience. Experience comes from bad judgment."

- There is an interface between mentoring, professionalism and career development.

- Mentoring is part of being a good leader

- There is a difference between coaching and mentoring.

- Coaching is a process where the coach works with an individual to identify or suggest ways of changing performance to improve results.

- Coaching usually is focused on developing individuals within their current job or position.

- Precepting means showing someone else how to perform your role, and is a key job retention strategy.

- A preceptor's responsibilities include role model, facilitator, educator, and evaluator.

- The role of the preceptor is crucial to the success of the new employee or student nurse.

- Organization culture must value and support the role by providing a formalized structure for the process.

Discussion Questions:

1. Define and explain mentoring.

2. Define and explain coaching.

3. Compare and contrast the differences between coaching and mentoring.

4. Explain the role of preceptor and why it is important to new healthcare workers.

Case Studies:

1. Carol is a middle manager in a community hospital. She noticed a respiratory therapy student crying in the nursing station, with a textbook open next to her. Carol approached the student and asked what was wrong. The student said "I am overwhelmed and I don't understand arterial blood gas values. I am going to fail!" How should Carol handle this student. Why? What should Carol be sure not to do? Why? If this was you as a student, how would you want to be treated?

2. Patricia lectured a lot on healthcare leadership. After a recent conference, an attendee came up to Patricia and asked if Patricia would mentor her. What should Patricia say? Do? How should she follow up?

WORKPLACE TRANSITION

Chapter 8
Instructor Guide

CHAPTER 8. WORKPLACE TRANSITION

Chapter Objectives:

1. Identify key workplace transitions

2. Explain being sidelined in your career

3. List three strategies to use if you experience a layoff/RIF.

4. List 4 items to consider if you are the person laying someone else off.

5. Explain what to do if you are terminated.

6. Explain the difference between termination and layoff.

7. Explain professional malaise and how to manage it

Key terms

Transition	return to work	transition management
Sidelined	outplacement	
RIF	termination	
Layoff	professional malaise	

Entering the Healthcare Workforce after Taking Time Off

- It is not uncommon take time off to have children or care for an elderly parent and return to the workforce when children are older.

- It is natural to feel awkward about getting back into the work environment.

- RELAX and have faith in your abilities. Remember, you had what it takes and that hasn't changed.

- If you look, sound and act confident and professional, most employers will believe you are hirable.

- Don't apologize for taking the time off

- Expect that employers will ask tough questions about your job gaps.

- Look at the questions as a chance to prove your mettle.

- Don't second guess your skills or credibility.

- Update your knowledge and find a way to practice your skills.

- Ask about being assigned a preceptor for assistance with getting your skills up to speed.

- Specialty healthcare tasks are a bit like bike riding…they come back as soon as you start pedaling and use them.

- Specialty skills are always in demand, and never more so than in a shortage.

- You can make a strong positive impression on potential employers before they every see your resume.

- Talking to strangers is a *good* idea when it comes to career development.

- Bring business cards with your contact information,

- Write a thank you note if someone provides you with a lead or other assistance.

- You will need to have basic computer literacy

- Informational interviews give you a chance to interview an individual in a role you are interested in

- When you are re-entering the workforce after time off, you may want to seek professional advice as to how to set up your resume to best highlight your past experience and skills.

- If you are a nurse, you may also wish to enroll in a nursing refresher/reentry program

When You Get Sidelined in your Career

- Do you feel increasingly out of the loop at work and seem to be watching the work process going on around you?

- Employees can be sidelined and pushed out of the mainstream without being aware it is happening.

- Organizations will only tolerate an employee out of the mainstream for a short period of time before the employee is terminated of laid off.

- The perception of realizing that one is on the outside comes so gradually it may be almost imperceptible until an event makes it plain to all.

- Hanging back, withdrawing from the craziness or just hiding out in your work space should be warning signs that you are approaching burnout or your problems are visible to others,

- You need to take action quickly–don't kid yourself about what is happening.

- The longer the inaction is observed, the fewer the choices.

- Don't put yourself in the position of having your job eliminated due to lack of productivity or inability to work with others.

Layoffs/Reduction in Force

- The scenarios for layoffs are always tough.

- No matter how it is presented, being laid off always comes as a personal blow. As a veteran of four layoffs myself, I know just how bad it feels.

- You can get what you deserve.

- You can ensure that you get maximum severance pay and benefits, as well as favorable references from your current employer.

- Take a deep breath and prepare to be successful at being out of a job.

- Don't take the layoff personally

- Don't lash out or try to get even

- Don't burn any bridges, as you may need them later.

- Leaving gracefully is a skill that will last much longer than the immature antics you can do when angry.

- Severance pay, references and benefit status are the most important issues to consider with a layoff.

- If possible, try not to discuss severance at that first notification meeting.

- Delaying the discussion will give you a chance to deal with your emotions and be able to think and negotiate clearly.

- Document as much as you possibly can about the lay-off meeting.

- Be sure to meet with someone from the human resources department.

- Ask about outplacement assistance.

- If you have outplacement services, use them

- Ask about references. Find out exactly who will be providing your reference information and what will be said.

- Make any requests about written and verbal references during the severance negotiation meeting.

- Negotiate as much as you can for severance pay.

- Ask for twice as much as you think you can get. You can always back down, but you can never ask for

- Most job searches these days take about 3 to 6 months, or longer in a poor economy

- Apply for unemployment insurance/benefits as soon as you can.

- Tell everyone you know that you are looking for work. As much as you want to keep the layoff private, the word leaks out anyway.

- networking with your colleagues can lead you to a new job.

- Compile a list of professional references.

- Never place someone on your reference list without asking their permission first.

- Remember that asking someone to be a reference means that they will put their reputation on the line in recommending you. Make sure you use it wisely.

- Be sure to keep your resume updated.

- Have business cards printed.

- Keep your interview skills polished.

- During the stressful time after a layoff, take good care of yourself.

- Don't take the first job you find because you are scared you won't get another offer.

- Do an honest self-assessment about your life, the type of job you want and your personal and professional goals.

- Find a job that is a good fit into your life.

- Layoffs can be a blessing in disguise!

If you are the person doing the reduction in force/lay off

- It is a gut-wrenching experience to downsize and reduce staff positions

- There are two sets of people affected by the layoff decision. Those who stay and those who go.

- People that leave the organization through layoffs are called the layoff victims. Those who are left in the organization are the layoff survivors.

- Often, the survivors have as many issues (if not more) than the victims.

- There is increased stress, decreased productivity, increased costs and overtime and changed workflows.

- People who survive a layoff can feel many emotions:

- It is critical to manage a layoff kindly and effectively.

- The backlash to a layoff handled poorly will last for years.

- Maintain the dignity of both the layoff victims and the survivors.

- Look at alternatives to layoffs including voluntary retirement, pay freezes, full time changed to part time status, etc.

- Layoff interventions must be planned and implemented prior to the layoffs and immediately after they occur.

- Keeping layoffs secret may not be a good plan.

- The longer the advance notification of a layoff is, the better employees can face and manage anxiety.

- Advance notice is almost always helpful.

- It is neither kind nor ethical to withhold that notice for other than strictly legal reasons.

- Remember that the most important resources are time and coaching.

- The most important tools to manage a layoff are education and communication.

- Recovery from a layoff must be managed from the top.

- Being proactive and empathetic, you can improve the organizational results over the long term.

- The most important tools to manage a layoff are education and communication.

If you are doing layoffs and remaining in the facility, remember

- Communication is everything

- Flood the survivors with information in all forms

- Use open communication, not controlled or contrived

- Tell the truth

- Never say never

- Explain the rationale and perception of fairness about the layoff and selection strategies

- Be visible as a manager on all your units and in areas of responsibility

- Be empathetic and share feelings

- Be authentic-not controlled or worried about "image"

- Identify the caretaking services offered to layoff victims-severance, outplacement and talk about those with the layoff survivors

- Lead with your heart first, then your head

- Remember, managing a layoff is more like managing a funeral than a financial situation

- Maintain the dignity of both victims and survivors

Turner Layoff Check List©

1. Don't panic

2. Remember, this is not disciplinary.

3. Don't get angry with your supervisor or the person who tells you.

4. Don't discuss severance at the first meeting. If possible, reschedule when you are not in shock.

5. Create a resume and keep it up to date.

6. Document as much as you can about your layoff meeting. Take notes during the meeting or write all you can remember as soon as you leave the meeting.

7. Meet with Human Resources (HR) to review your current benefit status and sign up for COBRA.

8. Ask for outplacement service, especially in lieu of severance.

9. Negotiate hard for severance pay. The rule of thumb is one week per year of service. However, most HR managers feel guilty about layoffs, so use this to your advantage. Ask for twice what you think you can get.

10. Don't sit on your severance monies as if they will last forever.

11. Clarify that your reference will document a reduction in force (RIF) not a termination.

12. Apply quickly for unemployment; it takes time to activate.

13. Leave the same day and take all your belongings. It is too painful to come back later.

14. Don't take hospital property or erase computer files. It may harm your chances of a good reference later on.

15. Ask for written references from Human Resources and your supervisor.

16. Keep an updated list of professional references.

17. Tell *everyone* you are looking for a job.

18. Keep in contact with colleagues.

19. Do not burn your bridges by publicly complaining about your previous employer. You never know who is sitting behind you in a restaurant or is in the next bathroom stall!

20. Take special care of yourself and try to use what you have the most of: TIME!

21. Review books and articles on resume writing, interviewing, career choices,

22. Remember you are not what you do!

Adapted from *American Association of Critical Care Nurses Transitions in Healthcare* curricula, 1996.

Original Source: Turner Healthcare Associates, 1994©

If you are Terminated from your Position

- Termination is traumatic.

- Sometimes it is totally unexpected.

- Most terminations occur after several counseling meetings and all other options to resolve the performance have been attempted.

- Being terminated from your position usually means you will not receive any severance pay.

- You will likely receive all earned sick and vacation time in your final check.

- You are often escorted from the building.

- The usual termination process involves a confidential meeting between you, your manager and a representative from Human Resources. If you are in a bargaining unit and represented by a union, you have the right to have a union representative at the meeting.

- Keep in mind that signing documents does not imply agreement with the circumstances, only receipt of the document.

- Ask about a grievance procedure, it should be reviewed at that time.

- Take everything with you, as it will be difficult to return.

- Being terminated from a position is a traumatic event.

- As tempting as it is to lash out at your manager, staff or human resources staff– *DON'T.*

- No matter what the circumstances, termination feels personal and many unpleasant feelings come up after it occurs.

- Maintain the dignity of an employee you terminate.

- Brainstorm to create summary sentences that you can say whenever anyone calls you.

- If the situation involves the news media and you are contacted, *DO NOT* (!!) make any statements that can be perceived as slanderous.

- Remember, *NOTHING* is ever off the record with any kind of reporter.

- Avoid writing letters to the newspaper, hospital administration or the board of directors complaining about your termination situation.

- Keep your dignity as much as possible.

- If you have a potential legal case, contact a lawyer directly and do not talk to your colleagues about any possibility of legal action.

- Do apply for unemployment insurance quickly, although in many cases of termination, you will not be eligible.

- Sometimes the reasons for your termination may have nothing to do with you.

- You are not what you do!

- Trying to hide a termination or lie about it is a bad idea.

- Show maturity and acknowledgement of your accountability for your actions.

- If your termination has legal ramifications or you are placed in a chemical diversion program, be honest about that as well.

- Employees who are honest about their mistakes and talk about what they learned from the termination do the best with transitioning into new roles.

- You can be terminated from a position and still be successful.

If you terminate an employee

- Be kind and compassionate.

- Pick a confidential and private location to talk with the employee being terminated.

- If the employee is to be escorted out of the unit, obtain the employee's personal belongings yourself, if possible.

- If you must share the vacancy of the position, do not state the employee was terminated in your communication with staff.

- Do not discuss the reasons or the circumstances about the termination with any employees other than human resources staff or supervisors that need to be made aware.

- Confidentiality is crucial, not only for the dignity of the employee, but for legal purposes.

- Be gentle and sincere.

- Your employee will be grateful and you may avoid a lawsuit.

Turner Termination Checklist©

1. Don't panic!

2. Don't get angry with your supervisor or the person who tells you of the termination.

3. Create a resume and keep it up to date.

4. Document as much as you can about your termination meeting. Take notes during the meeting or write all you can remember as soon as you leave the meeting. Keep copies of all materials you sign or receive.

5. If someone from Human Resources is not present at the termination meeting, ask to meet with them to review your current benefit status and sign up for COBRA *before* you leave the building.

6. Clarify what specific reference information will be provided to prospective employers.

7. Apply quickly for unemployment. You may not be eligible, but if you are, it takes time to activate.

8. Leave the same day and take all your belongings. It is too painful to come back later.

9. Don't take hospital property or erase computer files. It may harm your chances of a good reference later on.

10. Keep an updated list of professional references.

11. Tell everyone you are looking for a job. You can do this without divulging the termination.

12. Decide if you want to keep in contact with colleagues.

13. Do not burn your bridges by publicly complaining about your previous employer. You never know who is sitting behind you in a restaurant or is in the next bathroom stall!

14. Take special care of yourself and try to use what you have the most of: TIME!

15. Consider journaling about your termination experience. You can learn a lot from putting your experiences in writing.

16. Remember you are not what you do!

Turner Healthcare Associates, Inc. 2005©

Resigning your position

- You can resign and keep work relationships intact with just a little bit of proactive planning.

- Don't leave without any warning.

- Resignations should be made in writing, however leaving the letter for your manager to find on his/her desk is a last resort.

- Make an appointment with your manager to discuss your resignation.

- Inform your manager *before* you tell your coworkers.

- Finish out your shifts and maintain your dignity by not complaining during your last days at work.

- If you transfer out of a unit, but are not leaving the facility, you usually don't need to formally resign

- It is professional to tell your current manager where you are interested in transferring, and why.

- Most facilities have transfer deadlines and expect current managers and future managers to negotiate a transfer plan together.

- Do your best to be flexible and honor both managers' needs to have you working, if you can.

- If a going-away gathering is an option, participate graciously in the planning. If you do not want a gathering, say so early, so it doesn't appear that you are "raining on the parade" of your coworkers.

Negotiating a Raise

- Before you ask your boss for a raise, do your homework.

- Assess your performance from your supervisor's perspective.

- Schedule a meeting with your manager

- Use a percentage, not a dollar figure when voicing your raise request.

- In 2012, the national average for raises is 3% (Dickler, 2012

- If your raise is denied, be sure to say thanks anyway, and thank your boss for listening.

- Don't leave angry or make threats about resigning your position.

- Ask your boss about specifics on what you could do to be more successful about a raise in the future.

Professional Malaise

- Burnout implies inability to change the circumstances of your work perceptions. I prefer the term "professional malaise" because I believe the situation can be adjusted.

- This is not to be confused with compassion fatigue, which is much more serious.

- Compassion fatigue is the result of caring for others but not practicing self care (2012) and requires treatment for healing .

- Healthcare staff with professional malaise use more sick days, are less productive, depressed and often talk about how miserable they are.

- To avoid professional malaise, you must care for the caregiver just like the patient.

- Healthcare staff with burnout are easy to spot.

- Burnout symptoms affect your overall physical health.

- Healthcare facilities are starting to provide healthy choices for staff members right in the work place with smoking cessation and weight loss programs

- The ultimate choice to take better care of yourself rests with you.

- What have you done for yourself lately?

- Make sure you make time for yourself in your schedule.

- There is nothing wrong or unusual about having professional malaise.

- Professional malaise can be embraced and resolved.

- There are numerous reasons for developing professional malaise.

- Professional malaise is not a death sentence for your healthcare career.

- With recognition, support and an individual place to change your head space, you can move through professional malaise.

- You will come out of the experience as a better healthcare professional because of it.

Symptoms of professional malaise

- No accountability toward your professional specialty
- Experienced staff don't help you
- Other disciplines encroaching or dumping
- No one understands your professional care.
- You feel powerless and inflexible
- You feel unable to deal with work related conflicts
- You're not sure you have an organization that represents you
- You hate intra-professional infighting.
- You have no strategic plan or vision for you or your profession

Solutions for Professional Malaise

- There are ways to combat professional malaise in your life.

- It is important to admit you are having professional malaise.

- You need to make changes in your perceptions and in your work life.

- Dealing with professional malaise doesn't mean you have to change jobs.

- Does mean that you need to make changes in your work life.

- It is worthwhile to evaluate the root cause of your discomfort.

- Taking action to identify the problem means you will need to look at where you are currently in your career, as well as where you need to be for the future

- Create a new attitude.

- No more whining. If you whine, you are a victim. If you are a victim, you will feel powerless and perceive you can do nothing to change your circumstances. Nothing is further from the truth.

- During professional malaise, it can also help to find a mentor and/ or a coach.

Coping with Transition— Change your Headspace

- Healthcare staff routinely deal with lots of transition

- It is very difficult to deal with the emotional upheaval and moral angst that is included in the changes.

- *From Turmoil to Triumph,* by Mitchell Marks, highlights the change process that organizations must go through to be successful and deal with transition.

- Healthcare staff are great patient advocates, but not particularly good at advocating for themselves in a positive way.

- Marks identifies two types of transition as event driven and planned transformation.

- Event transition is triggered by an event, such as a merger, organizational redesign or downsizing.

- Planned transformation is a large-scale culture change with a cumulative series of changes that signal transition from an old way to new way of operating (Marks, 1994).

- Most healthcare professions have been exposed to both types of transition during the "restructuring and redesign" of the 'nineties.

- Individual staff experience planned transition every time a process or procedural change is made in a healthcare organization.

- Staff can also experience event transition when a facility is merged or sold.

- Industry-wide transition issues have happened in healthcare over the past two decades (managed care, prospective payment, work restructuring and redesign, patient safety mandates),

- There are numerous intra -professional issues that have never been resolved. Issues like what is the most appropriate level for entry into nursing practice, Associate Degree in Nursing or Bachelor's of Science in Nursing? Necessary education level for physical therapists? Dental assistants? These have been lingering unresolved for years.

- There is also an accelerated care expectation.

- This emphasis on time seems to ignore the fact that healing takes its own time, differs with each patient and cannot be regulated.

- The emphasis on time leads to healthcare based on task completion instead of caring for the patient as a whole person.

- The resulting chaos of this expectation has caused several states to legislate minimum safe nurse staffing regulations and ratios, and issues for other healthcare specialties.

- There are several stages that Marks identified and each healthcare worker goes through when dealing with change.

- Stage 1 = shock and fear

- Stage 2 = defensive retreat

- Stage 3 = acknowledgment of need for change

- Stage 4 = adaptation to change

These stages are similar to the three stages of change outlined by Edwin Lewin.

- Unfreezing = assessment of current environment and issues followed by shock and fear (this is where transition occurs)

- Changing = demonstrating new behaviors

- Refreezing = new behaviors become routine and the norm

Lewin believes that there are pushing and resisting forces for and against change that are working against each other at the same time.

If you make changes, you must go through the transition process before making the actual changes.

- It is common to resist change.

- It is also common for people to fear their own empowerment, which often represents change

- Managing change using organizational development skills

- Those building blocks of change are groups and teams.

- Organizations require collaborative environment, not competition between groups.

- Groups should lead decision making because they are the source of information.

- Organizations, groups and individuals manage affairs according to goals, not controls.

- Individuals and groups must participate in planning and implementing change.

- This will allow them to support what they help create.

- Managing change begins with the assessment process to determine how to proceed.

- The manager's job is to help staff deal with change.

- Managers may need help and training to deal with change, just like employees.

- changes cause conflict

- It is normal for any type of change to cause conflict, fear, confusion and an urge to return to the "old way" of doing things.

- Conflict management skills are necessary during the change process,

- Effective communication skills are vital

- Transition causes unsettling feelings:

- Can't have change without transition.

- You may find yourself initially resisting new headspace and professional philosophy.

- You may be doing things as coping strategies that are really personal sabotage

- You do not allocate resources (time, energy, money, passion) to the changes you wish to make

- You make a programmatic, flavor of the month change instead of a philosophic one.

- Career difficulties are an invitation for you to make changes.

- Managing transition is essential for a successful career-related change experience.

- Transition management is important in dealing with changes in your personal life as well.

- Recovery from the transition is essential to the process and means you must deal with the emotional realities of the transition.

- Going through transition is equivalent to the unfreezing step outlined in Lewin's change theory. (Marks, 1994)

- Professional transitions are opportunities for you to do things differently.

- Don't delegate or defer your career work

- *Remember who you are is not what you do!*

Professional Malaise Recovery

- Transition is a steady and constant state in healthcare these days.

- Transition is necessary for personal and career growth.

- After surviving a transition, most everyone sees it as a growth experience.

- No one can escape dealing with transition.

- You can determine how you deal with it.

- people change either by design or default. (Marks)

- You can approach to transition by purposefully creating strategies or you can do nothing and go with whatever happens.

- Healthcare staff tend to go with what they know.

- Familiarity is comfortable, but not always effective.

- If you want to do things differently, you need to change your plan for reacting.

- There are several ways to move through transition.

- You can retain old attitudes and change no behaviors OR

- Alter your mental model and settle into attitudes and behaviors inadvertently reinforced during your transition process OR

- You can alter your mental model and rely on attitudes and behaviors reinforced by the design of your personal transition management strategy.

- Change and transition will happen no matter what you do.

- If you decide to manage your transition, you can link your recovery plan to a personal quality improvement process

- Reject the temptation to create a "flavor of the month" change. It doesn't work in organizations and it won't work personally.

- In the absences of a plan, people go with what they know.

- You can survive and thrive during transition

- Motivate from the top down: first your head, then your heart

- Motivate from the inside-persuasion of your heart and mind, not just doing the behaviors.

- Be patient and empathetic with yourself and your resistance. This is HARD work!

- Remember that professional recovery and transition are personal imperatives to remain healthy and employed in a competitive (albeit fairly dysfunctional) industry

- You can create a new personal structure and philosophy by identifying your personal and professional direction.

- Consider writing your own mission statement for your life and career.

- Revitalize from the top down. First change your headspace, then your heart.

- You can resuscitate your spirit–something rarely achieved without transition.

Proactive Personal transition management

*Adapted from Marks organizational proactive transition management

P = Prepare yourself for a high level of activity

R = Rally yourself with a vision of a better you

O = Offer yourself transition training by learning how to deal with transition

A = Acknowledge your uncertainty and concerns

C = Communicate your plans and actions to others around you so they can support you

T = Tell others as much as you can about your transition management process

I = Involve others in managing your transition.

V = Visit with mentors and coaches.

E = Establish your personal safety net (self care, balanced life, career planning)

Turner Healthcare Associates, Inc. © 2001

Mastering Career Change

- You can achieve mastery of career change.

- The average person changes jobs six to eight times in a lifetime.

- You can survive and thrive during a job change.

- Job changes mean developing your problem-solving skills and refining and reframing your thinking.

- You are always more employable if you have a constant attitude of being willing to learn.

- Remember you are selling a product–YOU!

- Think of yourself as a valuable resource.

Turner Career Transition Model©

- The organizational change model relates to the same issues that individuals go through during transition.

- This is the process that every healthcare worker making a change should utilize for a successful career transition.

- When you experience a career transition, you start with deciding there needs to be a change made.

- Once you make the decision that a change is needed, determine the components related to actually making the change.

- You must deal with the emotional realities of the change you are pursuing.

- No matter how much we want to change, we will have sadness for what will no longer be.

- Allow yourself grieving and "hang" time.

- If you don't deal with the emotional realities or do any grieving, you may remain stuck in the same spot for a long time or be overwhelmed when you do make a change.

- Identify the processes and systems you need to put in place to make the change.

- Evaluate any resistance you have to creating these plans.

- Resistance to change is caused by failing to grieve and deal with the emotional realities of leaving the old behaviors.

- Resistance can be indicative of failing to create a good plan to make the transition.

- Resistance isn't bad-it is a signal to you that you may have forgotten one or more steps in the transition process, or you may be making a change you are not ready to make.

- Don't ignore your feelings of resistance.

- Allow yourself some adjustment time.

- "Hang" time becomes very valuable and allows you to adapt more easily to the transition process.

- Once you have embraced the transition, you can begin embracing the new change as a way of life.

- Once you are comfortable with the new norm, you have completed the transition process.

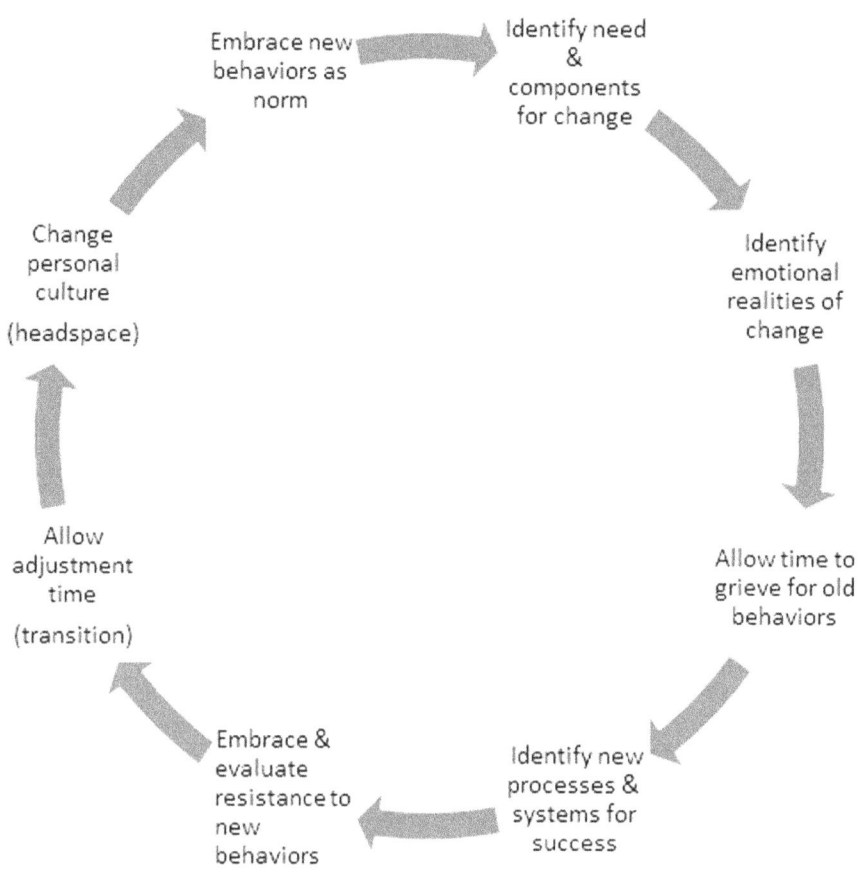

Turner Career Transition Model©

Turner Healthcare Associates, Inc. 1998©

Discussion Questions:

1. What are some of the key workplace transitions?

2. What does it mean to be sidelined in your career

3. What strategies would you use if you experience a layoff/RIF? Why?

4. What items/issues will you consider if you are the person laying someone else off? Why?

5. Explain what to do if you are terminated.

6. Explain the difference between termination and layoff.

7. Explain professional malaise and how to manage it.

Case Studies:

1. Melody was a former AA degree NICU RN. She had worked in NICU until she had her own children. She now worked in a clerical role at an aerospace company, but wanted to go back to nursing. As a fellow worker, she asks you for advice. What would you tell her as strategies? Why?

2. Karen worked as an ED clerk. She was smart, efficient and did great work. She made a joke to a Hispanic employee and everyone laughed. The employee looked sad but said nothing. The next day Karen came to work and was terminated from her job. What happened? Why? What should Karen do now? When she looks for another job?

YOUR EVOLVING CAREER

Chapter 9
Instructor Guide

CHAPTER 9. YOUR EVOLVING CAREER

Chapter Objectives:

1. Identify and explain the 5 usual functions of healthcare workers regardless of specialty.

2. Explain the difference between being a knowledge worker and a technical worker.

3. Explain the method of dealing with an angry patient or co-worker.

4. Identify assertive communication style and why it is effective.

5. List and explain the different types of power and why they are necessary in the healthcare workplace.

6. List 4 myths of use of power.

7. Explain conflict and identify issues related to experiencing it.

Key terms

Conflict management	dealing with angry staff or patients
Power myths	types of power
Assertive style	knowledge vs. technical worker
Advocate	

Professional Healthcare Roles

There are five usual functions of a healthcare worker, no matter what the specialty or role is. These functions include:

- Care provider– demonstrates skills in specific specialty, and appropriate communication skills

- Teacher– demonstrates knowledge of basic principles of the teaching-learning process within their specialty. Identifies clients' learning needs, capabilities and limitations, selection of appropriate information, material and strategies.

- Advocate– can state clients' rights and responsibilities as healthcare consumers, and identifies any issues between the clients and provider's perceptions of healthcare needs. May participates in client care conferences communicating clients' needs.

- Professional– demonstrated knowledge of the standards/criteria of competent performance and scope of professional specialty practice. Access own capabilities, limitations and accept accountability for actions. Establish goals for achieving professional growth.

- Supervisor– coordinate care of clients' with other healthcare specialties to achieve care outcomes and the provision of cost-effective, quality based services.

(*adapted from American Association of Colleges of Nursing 5 roles of nursing, 1998)

- There are other additional functions that every healthcare worker must exhibit in the workplace to be successful.

- Being indispensable is easier than it sounds.

- Focus your time on enhancing your skills, improving competencies and cultivating new ones.

Dealing with Angry Patients and Coworkers

- It is crucial to resist the impulse to get angry.

- Be quiet and listen to the co-worker.

- Upset people want to be heard more than anything else.

- Try not to plan what you are going to say back to them while they are talking. This interferes with your ability to listen.

- Don't jump in and answer right away; wait until they stop talking.

- Wait silently for a few seconds before you respond.

- Resist the urge to tell them that they shouldn't feel the way they do.

- Feelings are valid even when you don't agree.

- If you have made a mistake, acknowledge that you have done so, and apologize.

- Many times, anger is based on misperceptions and miscommunications.

- Wait until you are both calm to talk about the situation.

- It is appropriate to recognize feel, express and accept your own anger.

Try not to speak while you are angry

Assertive Communication

- Assertive communication is used for making and refusing requests, giving and receiving recognition and giving and receiving criticism (2012)

- It is common to have some anxiety and fear when considering use of an assertive style of communication.

Using Power for Managing Conflict

- Power is one of the most important job skills you can utilize.

- Power is not necessarily related to a position in an organization.

- Power is defined as the ability to control, influence or act.

- Authority is defined as the legitimate power granted to an individual by an organization. Power is vested in a position.

- Leadership is the relationship between two or more people in which one influences the other toward accomplishing a goal without legitimate power. (Bernard and Walsh, 1996)

- When you use power well, you can influence many events and processes in your workplace.

- There are several different types of power, as defined in management texts.

  - Personal power is the ability to link the outer capacity for action with the inner capacity of reflection.

  - Organizational power is the ability to accomplish goals through others within an organization.

  - Executive power is the use of personal persuasion and influence to motivate others.

  - Legitimate power is given to individuals based on their position in an organization. This leads to those individuals having designated authority.

  - Reward power is the power to provide distribution of rewards.

  - Coercive power is the ability to administer punishment, or the opposite of reward.

  - Expert power is earned by an individual with expert knowledge and skills in a certain area or industry.

  - Referent power is the ability to have influence over another based on respect and admiration.

- Managers need both power (all of the types) and authority to be effective.

- Healthcare workers often see power as bad or negative, but it is actually a neutral force.

- People who tend to feel powerless often display the inability to accomplish a goal.

- There are several myths about power. These include:

MYTH	*REALITY*
Power is bad	Power is neutral
Power is a goal	Power is a means to accomplish goals
Powerful people are ruthless	Powerless people are ruthless
Power can be given to others	Power must be earned or assumed
It is wrong or bad to want power	Power to accomplish goals can reduce stress and frustration

- The use of power also may cause conflict.

- Conflict is inevitable in life and at work

- Many healthcare workers are uncomfortable with conflict because they have had no training to deal with it.

- Conflict can make individuals and groups feel scared and powerless.

- Dysfunction organizations usually have lots of unresolved conflict.

- Before resolution of conflict can begin, the cause of the conflict must be identified.

- Conflict is over-feared and undervalued.

- Many healthcare workers are ineffective in managing conflict.

- Most healthcare workers would rather avoid conflict altogether than deal with whatever issue causes the tension.

- For the healthcare profession as a whole, conflict has often been avoided or glossed over and not dealt with. This has caused many formidable and difficult issues to be endlessly debated but never resolved.

- Conflict exists when two or more parties (individuals, groups or organizations) differ with regard to facts, opinions, beliefs, feelings, drives, needs, goals, methods, values or anything else.

- Disagreement between groups about their goals can create conflict

- Most organizational structures cause conflict to occur.

- Change almost always causes conflict.

- Conflict can resolve differences, clarify issues, and promote unity when managed effectively.

- To avoid conflict is to eliminate the possibility of defining goals, discussing issues, and designing a unifying philosophy about the issue.

- Conflict in and of itself is not bad. It creates tension and makes people feel uncomfortable.

- Conflict does enhance advocacy.

- There are two ways to deal with conflict.

- Conflict resolution seeks a solution that completely satisfies all parties involved in the conflict.

- The more common way to deal with conflict is through conflict management, which implies a conscious effort to deal with the conflict as well as the issue and control the problem.

- While difficult, it is much easier in the long run to deal with conflict head on.

- Not dealing with conflict is the single most limiting factor in resolving healthcare issues at both the local and national levels.

- We could be so much more powerful in dealing with healthcare social policy issues if the professionals were willing to "get down and dirty" to resolve its differences before airing its dirty laundry and splintered decisions in public.

- Conflict will always have to co-exist with healthcare.

- Resolving conflict takes a strong stomach and the willingness to be uncomfortable.

- Healthcare workers need to stop being afraid of conflict and start learning to use it.

Discussion Questions:

1. Explain the 5 usual functions of healthcare workers regardless of specialty, and provide an example of each in your specialty.

2. Explain the difference between being a knowledge worker and a technical worker. Why does it matter?

3. Demonstrate a method of dealing with an angry patient or co-worker.

4. Identify/role play assertive communication style and why it is effective. Samples of an assertive communication style are those that describe the situation or behavior e.g. "when you…." and expresses your reactions or feelings about it "I feel…" You would also use an assertive style to specify the change that you want to occur, e.g. "I want you to…" Assertive style also allows you to identify common goals or outcomes, e.g. "if that happens, then…." or "if you do this, then…."

5. Explain the different types of power and why they are necessary in the healthcare workplace.

6. Explain the concept of power and list 4 myths and realities when using power.

7. Explain conflict and identify issues related to experiencing it.

8. Discuss and explain an issue causing conflict within your healthcare specialty and potential resolution ideas.

Case Studies:

1. Sarah was a new manager in a community hospital. She had been in her role less than a year. A physician came up to her, clearly upset, and started screaming at her about a patient whose lab work was not yet in the chart for his review. How should Sarah respond to the MD? Why?

2. Betsy was a chief nurse executive of a large healthcare organization. She routinely told half-truths or untruths to her staff. She made a point of critiquing leadership styles of her staff in public locations. She routinely sat with the CEO of the organization. You are a staff member who works for Betsy. What should you about her, if anything?

3. Lori is a CEO of a community hospital, part of a large healthcare system. Lori routinely criticized individuals in public meetings with her managers and directors. One day she stated she would "kill anyone that doesn't comply with a rule." How would you respond as a member of the management team? If you were an employee she criticized? Why?

PROFESSIONAL ADVOCACY

Chapter 10
Instructor Guide

CHAPTER 10: PROFESSIONAL ADVOCACY

Chapter Objectives:

1. Define professional advocacy and explain why it is important.

2. List 4 ways to be a professional advocate.

3. List 8 characteristics of remarkable employees.

4. Compare and contrast embellishment vs. integrity.

5. Explain who is responsible for healthcare worker retention and why.

6. List 4 retention strategies for healthcare workers in your specialty and why they might be effective.

7. Identify key survival strategies during turbulent times.

8. List 3 risks and 3 rewards for using survival strategies

Key terms

Political advocacy   professional advocacy
Remarkable employee   Integrity
Retention   Nurturing young workers
Survival strategies   Professional networking

Key concepts

- Nurture those who come after you.

- Feed the machine.

- Be a healthcare worker 24/7.

- Let go of old issues.

- Cultivate your experiences and skills.

- Become a lifelong learner.

- Use staff to their maximum potential.

- Nurture yourself emotionally and spiritually.

- Be a Remarkable Employee

- Have integrity

- Don't embellish

- Utilize survival strategies: there are risks and rewards for doing so

- Healthcare means being of service to others

- Graciousness is Mandatory

- Abuse of any sort is a very serious issue and should not be tolerated, especially in the healthcare workplace

- Physician abuse of healthcare staff is a workplace retention issue.

- Networking with other professionals is a process of creating links to obtain information, influence and power.

- Knowing a connector is valuable to your career and using them well is priceless!

- Networking is a long term strategy for professional and career advancement

- Many healthcare issues that affect our communities are also social policy issues.

- Healthcare workers are in a unique position to educate politicians about health issues and affect change.

Discussion Questions:

1. Define professional advocacy and explain why it is important.

2. List 4 ways to be a professional advocate.

3. List 8 characteristics of remarkable employees.

4. Explain who is responsible for healthcare worker retention and why.

5. List 4 retention strategies for healthcare workers in your specialty and why they might be effective.

6. Identify key survival strategies during turbulent times.

7. List 3 risks and 3 rewards for using survival strategies

8. explain the concept of networking and why it is important

9. list 5 activities that are part of networking

10. explain the purpose and value of joining a professional organization.

11. Discuss the value of political advocacy.

Case Studies:

1. Use Yahoo CEO case study to discuss embellishment vs. integrity, risks and rewards of both http://articles.latimes.com/2012/may/14/business/la-fi-yahoo-thompson-resigns-20120514

2. Bev is an operating room nurse with 30 years experience. During a surgical procedure, the surgeon became upset at the way Bev was passing him instruments. He screamed at her, in the OR with other staff present, and then proceeded to throw a surgical light (30 inches in diameter, on a stand) at her arm. She had her elbow broken in 3 places, spent 3 months in the hospital and was unable to return to work. She is now on permanent disability. How should the hospital handle the surgeon? The medical staff ? Bev? What are their options? Why?

Reference Articles on abuse: http://www.findarticles.com/p/articles/mi_m0FSL/is_3_74/ai_80159514

http://www.usnews.com/usnews/health/articles/020617/archive_021640.htm

http://xnet.kp.org/permanentejournal/winter04/pal.html

http://healthcare.monster.com/nursing/articles/verbalabuse/

http://www.nursingcenter.com/library/JournalArticle.asp?Article_ID = 278949

http://www2.nurseweek.com/Articles/article.cfm?AID = 14548

http://educate.crisisprevention.com/WorkplaceViolence.html?code = ITG006SCWE&src = Pay-Per-Click&gclid = CIHuwJGTq7ACFccBRQodT09-XQ

http://www.lni.wa.gov/safety/research/files/bullying.pdf

http://counselingoutfitters.com/vistas/vistas05/Vistas05.art62.pdf

http://www.workplacebullying.org/individuals/problem/definition/

http://suite101.com/article/emotional-abuse-in-the-workplace-a73977

http://educate.crisisprevention.com/WorkplaceViolence.html?code = ITG006SCWE&src = Pay-Per-Click&gclid = CMLmtvyTq7ACFQF6hwodSUVVVg

CREATING YOUR HEALTHCARE FUTURE

Chapter 11 Instructor Guide

CHAPTER 11. CREATING YOUR HEALTHCARE FUTURE

Chapter Objectives:

1. Identify 3 future trends in healthcare and how they will affect your specialty.

2. List two environmental factors that impact your healthcare practice and specialty.

3. List the goals of the triple aim initiative.

4. Identify the components of the healthcare framework in the future.

5. Define and explain an ACO.

Key terms

Triple aim initiative	Medicare
diversity	ACO
aging	healthcare framework
technology	self-governance
workforce	healthcare architecture
healthcare financing	retention
healthcare structures	

Future Trends in Healthcare

- "It is easy to come up with new ideas; the hard part is letting go of what worked for you two years ago, but will soon be out of date."

- the architecture of healthcare has been based on a foundation of patient advocacy and achieving maximum beneficial outcomes for each patient.

- The framework of care for patients included specialization of services, fragmented components of care, a narrow focus with minimum flexibility and an "us vs. them" mentality..

- Several environmental factors are impacting the future of healthcare practice. These factors include:

1. Diversity-changing demographics in states' populations, the diversity of the healthcare workforce and public views of healthcare and healthcare policy issues.

2. Aging-impact of an aging population on healthcare systems, financing of healthcare and demand for some healthcare professions (nursing, pharmacists) aging nursing workforce, and the development of new healthcare services.

3. Technology-the impact of global technology on healthcare roles and practice.

4. Workforce-challenges in healthcare workforce supply, demand, education and role definition.

5. Healthcare financing-increasing costs and financing impact on delivery systems, community based health programs and healthcare practice roles.

6. New structures required to meet future needs e.g. Accountable Care Organizations, part of the Obama Healthcare Reform Act currently under review in the Supreme Court. Accountable Care Organizations (ACOs) are groups of doctors, hospitals, and other health care providers, who come together voluntarily to give coordinated high quality care to their Medicare patients.

- Patient advocacy and maximum beneficial care outcomes will continue to drive the way care is provided.

- The framework that healthcare must build for future practice must be focused on specific professional roles as well as integration of services, a community wide focus, flexibility and cross training of staff, commitment to lifelong learning and professional development, the mindset of "us helping them" and one focused, professional voice with which care practices are changed to meet the needs of all patients.

- Accountable Care Organizations are designed to provide consistent care of high quality to a specific group of patients while controlling costs.

- Triple Aim Initiative (2007). This initiative was designed to:

- Improve the health of the population

- Enhance patients' experience of care including quality, access and reliability

- Control or reduce cost of care

- To evaluate how to achieve this, certain high performance healthcare delivery organizations were studied.

- ACOs are a dramatic change for current healthcare delivery.

- Hospitals, skilled nursing, long-term acute care, hospice and mental health facilities can all be part of ACOs as well as physicians, independent practitioners and outpatient facilities.

- To achieve this new architecture and framework for healthcare practice, there are additional changes that will be seen across the profession within the next 20 years.

- The healthcare workplace will be transformed.

- Retention will be the healthcare focus instead of recruitment, especially as boomers retire.

- The future for healthcare will require specific leadership strategies.

- The utilization of evidenced based practice, outcomes focused measurements for patients, and research based practice will be commonplace.

- Most healthcare professions will work in a self-governed workforce in a shared governance model within healthcare organizations.

- Labor unions will have less impact on staffing

- There will be social and community activism around health and policy related issues.

- The role of the registered nurse in the future will be as a director and coordinator of care, not just a task provider.

- Many healthcare roles will have an expanded practice with a redirected focus towards wellness.

- Healthcare will function in a community-based model using a case management approach to care along the health-illness continuum

- These changes will require great transition management skills.

Creating your Personal Healthcare Future

- It is easy to be passionate about a profession that gives you so many job options and career choices. Healthcare forces you to be the best you can be, no matter what your role.

- Lifelong learning throughout your healthcare career will put you on the path to excellence.

- Life is about learning, and learning is about change.

- Each one of us has a responsibility as a professional to secure care for our nation's population as well our profession's future.

- We hold the keys to the solutions to change systems and processes.

- Use your influence to enhance care and your profession in a positive way.

- Using your healthcare influence to enhance care is really about being a leader in society and using leadership skills.

- Generate a sense of purpose in your organization that honors your profession and the patients you care for.

- Support the renaissance of healthcare professions by mentoring kindly those who come after you, and showing them the ways of the future.

- Demonstrate the qualities of a winner as you plan your career goals and your future.

Discussion Questions:

1. Identify 3 future trends in healthcare and discuss how they will affect different healthcare specialties.

2. Discuss environmental factors that impact your healthcare practice and specialty.

3. Discuss whether the Triple Intiative is a good idea and why.

4. Discuss the environmental factors' effects on healthcare and determine potential ramifications.

5. Discuss the new healthcare framework for the future.

6. Discuss the effect of ACOs in your geographic area.

7. Discuss what Warren Bennis believes people want from their leaders.

Case Studies:

1. Henry is a hospital CEO. He is the CEO of the biggest hospital in a small healthcare system. He is well respected and enjoys the popularity that comes with working at a facility for 25 years in both clinical and administrative roles. He has been the CEO for 15 years. His qualities include finance skills, "clinical mindset", a strong relationship with board members and strong community relationships. His leadership style and characteristics include micro-management, need to approve every document prior to it being sent by every manager, lack of trust in key players, changing strategic direction frequently. Will he be successful in the next ten years? Why or why not?

2. You are asked by your boss to spearhead the development of an ACO in your community. Who will you meet with? Who are your stakeholders? Why? What steps will you take to set up this group?

3. What does the reading on the next page mean to you? Why?

THE WINNER

The Winner is always a part of the answer.
The Loser is always a part of the problem.
The Winner always has a program.
The Loser always has an excuse.
The Winner says, "Let me do it for you."
The Loser says "That's not my job"
The Winner sees an answer for every problem.
The Loser sees a problem for every answer.
The Winner says it may be difficult, but it's possible.
The loser says it may be possible, but it's too difficult.
A Winner listens.
A Loser waits until it's his turn to talk.
When a Winner makes a mistake, he says "I was wrong."
When a Loser makes a mistake, he says. "It wasn't my fault."
A Winner says "I'm good, but not as good as I could be."
A Loser says, "I'm not as lots of other people."
A Winner feels responsible for more than his job.
A Loser says "I only work here."

-Author unknown

HEALTHCARE CAREER GUIDE REFERENCES

1. Association of California Nurse Leaders, *ACNL Resource Guide for Political Action*, 1995.

2. Cowles, Luke, "First Impressions", <u>Advance for Nurses</u>, March 7, 2005 p.23

3. Mehallow, Cindy, "Nursing Careers Beyond the Bedside" http://featuredreports.monster.com/nursing05/nonclinical/

4. Mehallow, Cindy,"Nursing Careers Beyond the Hospital" http://featuredreports.monster.com/nursing05/nonhospital/

5. <u>Rossheim</u>, John "Nurses Who Teach" http://featuredreports.monster.com/nursing05/professorship/

6. <u>Malugani</u>, Megan "Up-and-Coming Nurse Niches" http://featuredreports.monster.com/nursing05/niches/

7. <u>Malugani</u>, Megan "Legal Nurse Consulting" http://featuredreports.monster.com/nursing05/legal/

8. Meyeroff, Wendy J. "Advance Your Nursing Career" http://featuredreports.monster.com/nursing05/advancedspecialties/

9. Worthington, Michael "Top 20 Recruiter Pet Peeves About Resumes", http://resumedoctor.com/

10. Gaffin, Norma Mushkat, "Recruiters' Top 10 Resume Pet Peeves" http://resume.monster.com/articles/petpeeves/

11. Lipow, Valerie, "Interviewing 101" http://hourlyandskilled.monster.com/retail/articles/retailinterviewing/

12. Barada, Paul W. , "How Do You Sell Yourself When You Don't Have Much to Sell?" http://content.monstertrak.monster.com/resources/archive/jobhunt/toughsell/

13. Voght, Peter "Measure Your Soft Skills Smarts" http://content.monstertrak.monster.com/resources/archive/jobhunt/softskills

14. Advance News magazine, "Advancing Your Career" htto://www.advanceweb.com

15. Versant RN Residency www.versant.org

16. Smith, Mike, "Beyond Competent", <u>Emergency Medical Services</u>, June, 2005, pg 42.

17. Hollander, Jim. Onboard medical facilities have cruise passengers covered. *Los Angeles Times,* Sunday , June 26, 2005, pg L3

18. Buerhaus P., Implications of an Aging Registered Nurse Workforce *JAMA*, June 14, 2000; vol. 83, no. 22.

19. Dick, Thom, *Listening: Defusing the Angry Employee* <u>Emergency Medical Services</u>, June, 2005 p. 28

20. Rundio, Al *Ten management pearls for success"* Nurseweek, 2005 Pathways to success, p 24-5.

21. McLinden, Steve, *Navigating Organizational Culture,* Nurseweek, 2005 Pathways to success, p 102-05.

22. Gates, Polly Rubano, Joan; *Executive Coaching or Mentoring: Which way should you go?* DirectLink Newsletter, Association of California Nurse Leaders, Fall 2004,p.1

23. Brownstein, M. *Coaching and Mentoring for Dummies,* Foster City; IDE Books Worldwide, Ind. (2000)

24. Lewin, K. *Group decision and social change,* In Newcomb, T, Hartely E. ed., *Readings in Social Psychology,* New York, Holt, Rinehart Winston, 1947

25. Turner, Susan Odegaard, *Nurses guide to managed care,* 1999, Aspen Publishers

26. Turner, Susan Odegaard, *Has the Restructuring of Registered Nursing Roles in Hospitals Been Successful?* doctoral dissertation , College of Business, Southern California University, 1998

27. Turner, Susan Odegaard , *Transitions in Healthcare Series*, American Association of Critical Care Nurses, 1996

28. Stern, C. *Kaiser Foundation Hospital Graduate Nurse Handbook of Job Searching Techniques*, 4th ed, Oakland, California, Kaiser Permanente Hospitals (1990)

29. Kennedy, M. M. "When your career is sidelined" *Executive Female*, *September*/October, 1996. 33-35

30. yourownrubyslippers.com

31. the transitionnetwork.org

32. coachfederation.com

33. Advisory Board Daily Briefing (2001, April 9) "Severe Nursing Shortage is Threat to Patient Care",

34. Allen, Jane E (2001, May 7) "U.S. Nurses Not Alone in Their Frustration," Los Angeles Times.

35. Brown, Steve, (2001, May 21) "Congress Spotlights Nursing Shortage, Rural Wage Index Workforce Issues", AHA News 37(20).

36. Buerhaus, P., Staiger, D.O., and Auerbach, D.I., (2000). "Implications of an Aging Registered Nurse Workforce" Journal of the American Medical Association, 283 (22), 2948-2987.

37. Buerhaus P. (2000, June 14) "Implications of an Aging Registered Nurse Workforce." Journal of the American Medical Association, 83 (22).

38. California Board of Registered Nursing (2009), Annual School Report,. Sacramento: author.

39. Coffman, J., Spetz, J., Seago, J.A., Rosenoff, E., O'Neil, E. (2001, January). Nursing in California: A Workforce Crisis. San Francisco: Workforce Initiative and the UCSF Center for the Health Professions.

40. Erwin J. (1999, March 29) "Aging Out? Will the Rising Age of O.R. Nurses Lead to a Shortage?" NurseWeek.

41. Fackelmann K. (2000, June 15) "Study Predicts Nursing Shortage" USA Today.

42. Hughes J. (2000, May 7) "Shortage in Profession Persists." Times Dispatch.

43. Russell G. (2000, April 21) "Nursing Schools See Enrollment Steadily Shrink", <u>Telegram Gazette</u>. RN Scope of Practice, <u>California Business and Professional Code, Section 2725.</u>

44. Ruiz M. (2000, Third Quarter) "Nursing Shortage" <u>Sigma Theta Tau International Honor Society of Nursing in Clinical Practice</u>. 2948-2954

45. "2000 National Sample Survey of Registered Nurses," <u>Health Resources and Services Administration,</u> author, .

46. Selis S. (2000, June) "Where Have All the Nurses Gone?" <u>Healthcare Business</u>. 3 (4), 65-70.

47. Buerhaus, Peter, changing demographics of nursing *Health Affairs* November 17, 2004.

48. DeRitis, S. New Opportunities within Healthcare Informatics, *Advance,* April 26, 2004, p. 31.

49. Dr. Phil (McGraw) Column, Oprah, June 2005. p. 31.

50. Gladwell, Malcolm ,*Tipping Point*, Little Brown, New York,2004

51. Noer, David "After the Pink Slips" *Executive Female,* July/ August, 1995 p.43-45.

52. Kaye, B.L., Jordan-Evan, S. (2002). <u>*Love 'em or lose 'em: Getting good people to stay*</u>. San Francisco, CA. Benett-Koehler Publishers.

53. Abrams, M (2002, March). "Employee retention and turnover: Holding managers accountable" *Trustee*. Chicago, 55 (3), T1.

54. Hugg, Alicia, "Forging Ahead", *Nurseweek,* July 4, 2005, p.8-10.

55. Steefel, L. "Survey shows first real positive workforce change", *Nurseweek*, July 4, 2005 p.15.

56. Bach, David "Get that Raise" *Working Mother,* September 2005, p. 52.

57. Lichtenberg, Ronna "Designing a future that fits" *More* July/ August, 2005 p. 60-64.

58. Merritt, Jennifer, "Get-Ahead Strategies You've Never Heard Before" http://reference.aol.com/onlinecampus/campusarticle?id=20050712200509990001

59. Thomas, D., 1994 "Five Ways to Run Your Career Like a business" *Executive Female*, November/December 37-40.

60. Hitt, M, Middlemist, R and Mathis, R, 1986, *Management concepts and effective practice,* 2nd ed. Houston, Texas, West Publishing.

61. Bernstein, A. and Craft-Rozen, S. "Why don't they just get it?" *Executive Female* March/April, 1995 p 33-7.

62. Beverly Health and Rehabilitation Services, Rancho Cordova, CA, *Supervisory Training Modules.*

63. Lyon, Mary "The ABCs of Pursuing Higher Education in Nursing", *Nurseweek Career Fair,* 1998.

64. Fischman, Josh **"Nursing Wounds",** *US News and World Report,* http://www.usnews.com/usnews/health/articles/020617/archive_021640.htm

65. Brzezicki, Lisa, "Caring for the Caregiver" *Advance for Nurses,* Southern California edition; August 22, 2005 p.9.

66. Mooney, Bette, "Resolving Conflicts" *Advance for Nurses,* Southern California edition, July 11,2005, p.15.

67. Bensing, K, "No Stone Unturned", *Advance for Nurses,* Southern California edition, August 8, 2005, p.11.

68. Goulette, Candy, "Under their Wings", *Advance for Nurses,* Southern California edition, June 13, 2005 p.38-9.

69. Johnson, James, "Warren Bennis, Chariman, The Leaderships Institute, *Healthcare Executive*, 1998 http://www.ache.org/pubs/hcexecsub.cfm

70. *Benefits of becoming a Magnet-designated facility* http://www.nursingworld.org/ancc/magnet/benes.html

71. Komisarjevskys, "Peanut Butter and Jelly Management: Tales from Parenthood Lessons for Managers" (Amacom, 2004).

72. Abrams, M (2002, March). Employee retention and turnover: Holding managers accountable. Trustee. Chicago, 55 (3), T1.

73. AONE. (2002, Sept.). Say what? What California nurses say about working, Nurseweek/AONE Study

74. Buckingham, M., Coffman, C. (~2001). First, break all the rules: What the world's greatest managers do differently. New York, NY. Simon & Schuster.

75. Robbins, Stephen, *Organizational behavior,* 7th ed. 1996, Prentice Hall.

76. Myss, Caroline, S*acred Contracts*, Three Rivers Press, New York, 2003

77. Stringer, Heather, "Turning Point" *Nurseweek*, August 29,2005, p. 12.

78. Deleonardi, Bette "Lifelong Learning," *Advance for Nurses,* September 5, 2005, p.17-22.

79. Warren, Rick *The Purpose Driven Life,* Zondervan, Michigan, 2002

80. https://www.cms.gov/Medicare/Medicare-Fee-for-Service-Payment/ACO/index.html?redirect=/ACO/.

81. http://www.bls.gov/emp/ep_table_103.htm

82. http://www.nhscareers.nhs.uk/atoz.shtml

83. http://www.bls.gov/oco/cg/cgs035.htm

84. http://explorehealthcareers.org/en/getting_started/is_a_health_career_right

85. http://www.ama-assn.org/go/alliedhealth

86. http://www.aamc.org/students

87. http://bhpr.hrsa.gov/

88. : http://www.caahep.org

89. http://www.bls.gov/ooh/

90. http://www.iom.edu/Reports/2001/Crossing-the-Quality-Chasm-A-New-Health-System-for-the-21st-Century.aspx

91. http://www.ihi.org/offerings/Initiatives/TripleAim/Pages/default.aspx

92. http://news.nurse.com/apps/pbcs.dll/article?AID = 2012104230004

93. http://benefitsattorney.com/modules.php?name = Content&pa = showpage&pid = 14

94. http://www.personalbrandingblog.com/develop-your-career-like-a-business/

95. http://www.lifecoaching.com/pages/life_coaching.html

96. http://currentnursing.com/nursing_theory/Patricia_Benner_From_Novice_to_Expert.html

97. http://entrepreneursuccesstools.com/2010/09/23/time-management-peter-drucker/

98. http://www.nwlink.com/~donclark/leader/leadcom.html ,2012

99. http://www.strategy-business.com/article/re00063?gko = ae079

100. Robbins, by Stephen P, Truth about managing people– FT Press, 2 edition (September 30, 2007)

101. http://www.teamtechnology.co.uk/tuckman.html

102. Marks, Mitchell From Turmoil to Triumph: New Life After Mergers, Acquisitions, and Downsizing,1994

103. http://money.cnn.com/2011/07/27/pf/employee_pay/index.htm

104. http://www.compassionfatigue.org/

105. http://managementhelp.org/personalproductivity/problem-solving.htm#guide

LIST OF ORGANIZATIONS AND WEB SITES

*This page needs some sort of disclaimer about the websites, listing here is not an endorsement, etc.

Organizations

American Nurses' Association	http://nursingworld.org
National League of Nursing	http://www.nln.org
The Forum on Health Care Leadership	http://www.healthcareforum.org
Bureau of Labor Statistics	http://www.bls.gov
American Hospital Association	http ://www.aha.org
American Organization of Nurse Executives	http://www.aone.org
American Association of Colleges of Nursing	http://aacn.nche.edu
Johnson /Johnson site	http://www.discovernursing.com
Monster.com	http://www.monster.com
Health Career information	http://www.healthprofessions.com
Health Career information	http://www.healthcareers.com
Visa Information	http://www.visalaw.com
Nursing Spectrum	http://www.nursingspectrum.com
National Student Nurses Association	http://www.nsna.org
Links to nursing web sites	http://www.nursezone.com
Johnson and Johnson Nursing site	http://www.choosennursing.com
The Forum on Health Care Leadership	http://www.healthcareforum.org
Bureau of Labor Statistics	http://www.bls.gov
Specialties certifications	http://www.nursingcertification.org
Political info on healthcare	http://www.healthvote.org
Nurse practitioners	http://www.aanp.org
Association of California nurse leaders	http: www.acnl.org
US Senate	http:www.senate.gov
US House of representatives	http:www.houseofrepresentatives.gov
US legislature	http://www.legislature.gov

Career Transition

The Transition Network ....http://www.thetransitionnetwork.org

Ruby Slippers .... http://www.yourownrubyslippers.com

International Coach Federation ....http://www.coachfederation.com

www.ingramcontent.com/pod-product-compliance
Lightning Source LLC
Chambersburg PA
CBHW081454170526
45166CB00008B/2430